Diagnosis and Management of
Respiratory Diseases

The *Diagnosis and Management* Series is intended to cover the major fields of medicine in its sub-specialties. The emphasis throughout is in providing practical guidance to the clinician presented with a diagnostic or management problem.

This book is the second edition of the *Diagnosis and Management of Respiratory Diseases*. In it, Dr G.K. Crompton has utilized his extensive clinical experience and his skills as a teacher. All the chapters have been rewritten and several new chapters have been added. The book provides a comprehensive account of the diagnostic features and the management of respiratory disorders. Each topic is set out clearly under separate headings and each chapter concludes with a summary of special points of emphasis. The style is disarmingly simple, and this conceals the fact that the book contains much more scientific information than might appear at first glance.

Although the book is designed primarily for the clinician faced with a problem, it is also of value to candidates preparing for a higher degree, especially the second part of the Membership Examination, and to other hospital doctors, general practitioners and senior students who require a concise review of the 'state of the art' in respiratory medicine.

J.F. Munro
Series Editor

Diagnosis and Management of Respiratory Diseases

GRAHAM K. CROMPTON

MB FRCPE
Consultant Physician, Respiratory Unit
Northern General Hospital, Edinburgh
Senior Lecturer in Medicine and Respiratory Diseases
University of Edinburgh

SECOND EDITION

BLACKWELL SCIENTIFIC PUBLICATIONS

OXFORD LONDON EDINBURGH
BOSTON PALO ALTO MELBOURNE

© 1980, 1987 by
Blackwell Scientific Publications
Editorial offices:
Osney Mead, Oxford, OX2 0EL
8 John Street, London, WC1N 2ES
23 Ainslie Place, Edinburgh, EH3 6AJ
52 Beacon Street, Boston
    Massachusetts 02108, USA
667 Lytton Avenue, Palo Alto
    California 94301, USA
107 Barry Street, Carlton
    Victoria 3053, Australia

First published 1980

Set by Colset Private Limited, Singapore
and printed and bound in
Great Britain by Billings and Sons
Ltd, London, Oxford and
Worcester

DISTRIBUTORS
USA
    Year Book Medical Publishers
    35 East Wacker Drive
    Chicago, Illinois 60601

Canada
    The C.V. Mosby Company
    5240 Finch Avenue East,
    Scarborough, Ontario

Australia
    Blackwell Scientific Publications
    (Australia) Pty Ltd
    107 Barry Street
    Carlton, Victoria 3053

British Library
Cataloguing in Publication Data

Crompton, Graham K.
    Diagnosis and management of respiratory
    diseases.——2nd ed.
    1. Respiratory organs——Diseases
    I. Title
    616.2   RC731

ISBN 0-632-01675-2

Contents

Preface

This book is a comprehensive account of the diagnostic features and management of respiratory diseases written in a didactic and concise form to enable the reader to gain quick access to the important information.

Each topic is set out clearly under a separate heading, and the chapters are summarized by special points of emphasis. The contents have been thoroughly revised and brought up to date; in particular, there is a new chapter on adult respiratory distress syndrome, and the chapters on bronchial asthma and pulmonary thromboembolic disease have merited special attention.

The book is a valuable aid for the clinician faced with a problem, and will be useful to candidates studying for higher degree, and to medical students and general practitioners who require a concise review of up-to-date knowledge of respiratory diseases.

Chapter 1
Clinical findings

Introduction

There are six common symptoms of respiratory disease. Cough and breathlessness are features of almost all respiratory disorders. However, by taking an accurate history of each individual symptom and its relationship to others it is often possible for the correct diagnosis to be suggested by the history alone. A likely diagnosis or short list of possible diagnoses should be formulated before physical examination and the presence, or absence, of abnormal physical signs can then be integrated with the history to produce a rational clinical diagnosis.

There are five common groups of bronchopulmonary disorders which are responsible for the vast majority of symptoms and abnormal physical signs. These are:

Simple infections
Tuberculosis
Tumours
Respiratory disorders secondary to cardiovascular disease
    Pulmonary oedema
    Pulmonary thromboembolic disease
Obstructive airways diseases.

If these common disease categories are considered in the assessment of all symptoms, abnormal physical signs and radiographic abnormalities, diagnosis is usually relatively straightforward in all but a few rare diseases.

Symptoms

The six common symptoms are:
    Cough
    Sputum
    Haemoptysis
    Breathlessness
    Wheeze
    Pleuritic chest pain.

Cough

Cough is the most frequent symptom of all and is a manifestation of almost all airways diseases and many pulmonary pathologies. Coughing involves a number of respiratory manoeuvres:

An initial inspiration.

Occlusion of the glottis by closure of the vocal cords.

Contraction of the respiratory muscles against the closed glottis to produce a positive pressure within the airways.

Rapid opening of the vocal cords to allow explosive exit of air (and secretions) from the trachea.

Hence the clinical characteristics of 'normal' cough can be altered by:

1   Inability to breathe in efficiently, e.g. weakness or paralysis of the respiratory muscles: feeble cough. Obstruction to the larynx or main airways: inspiratory croup or stridor.

2   Inability to close and open the glottis, e.g. left vocal cord paralysis: bovine cough. Laryngeal oedema: croup.

3   Inability to contract expiratory muscles efficiently against a closed glottis, e.g. polyneuritis, myasthenia gravis: feeble cough or inability to cough.

4   Inefficient explosive expiration — as well as respiratory muscle and vocal cord abnormalities the usually forceful release of air from the larynx can be impaired by diffuse airways obstruction — e.g. asthma, chronic bronchitis: ineffective paroxysms of coughing associated with expiratory wheeze.

Although most diseases cause cough which has no specific characteristics, valuable diagnostic information can be obtained from the history, such as the time cough is most troublesome, its duration and association with other symptoms. For instance, cough troublesome first thing in the morning after a good night's sleep suggests chronic bronchitis, whereas cough associated with wheeze in the middle of the night is more typical of asthma. Persistent distressing cough in an adult smoker must always raise the suspicion of bronchial carcinoma.

The association of sputum production with cough is obvious. A persistent unproductive or 'dry' cough in an adult could indicate bronchial carcinoma, and a productive or 'loose' cough of long duration and brought on by changes in posture is characteristic of bronchiectasis. In the early stages of infections of the respiratory tract cough is often unproductive.

Sputum

Sputum production is always indicative of disease. Some patients, especially children and women, cough up sputum but swallow it. Careful assessment of the appearance of sputum is extremely important and useful information can be obtained from estimating sputum volume. Viscosity varies considerably.

SPUTUM APPEARANCE

Sputum may be serous, mucoid, purulent or mucopurulent.

Serous sputum indicates excessive non-infected production of broncho-pulmonary secretion. Serous sputum is frothy or watery and is often described by patients in these terms — e.g. acute pulmonary oedema. A rare but frequently quoted cause of copious watery sputum is bronchioloalveolar cell carcinoma.

Mucoid sputum, often described by patients as clear, grey or white, indicates excessive secretion of bronchial mucus and is characteristic of chronic bronchitis. Because of the chronicity of symptoms production of mucoid sputum is often accepted as normal and may not be readily admitted.

Purulent and mucopurulent sputum.   Sputum containing leucocytes is a turbid yellow or green colour and in the vast majority of cases this indicates bacterial infection. Very rarely an abundance of eosinophils can produce 'purulent' sputum. Patients often use the terms 'yellow', 'green' or 'dirty' to describe purulent sputum, but care must be taken in the interpretation of 'dirty sputum' as this can merely be a description of inhaled soot by urban dwellers.

The estimation of the amount of pus in the sputum is a good clinical guide to the severity of bacterial infection and a reliable means of assessing response to treatment.

Offensive-smelling purulent sputum, often said to have a foul taste, usually means deep-seated bronchopulmonary infection, e.g. lung abscess and bronchiectasis. Occasionally jet black sputum (mela-noptysis) can be produced by patients with coalworker's pneumo-coniosis.

Other appearances.   Blood-staining of sputum must always be regarded as indicative of serious pathology (*see* Haemoptysis). Rusty or orange-coloured sputum occurs in pneumococcal infections.

SPUTUM VOLUME

Sputum volume varies tremendously in different pathologies and also in patients with the same disease. Large volumes of purulent sputum suggest bronchiectasis or lung abscess.

SPUTUM VISCOSITY

In general, mucoid sputum is more viscid than purulent. Patients with chronic bronchitis often have more difficulty in coughing up mucoid than purulent sputum. The sputum in asthma is characteristically viscid, and plugging of bronchi is a major complication of severe episodes. Some patients with asthma produce tubular casts of bronchi (*see* p. 60).

Haemoptysis

Coughing up blood must always be assumed to be of serious significance and always warrants appropriate investigation (Table 1.1). In many cases, however, no cause can be found. It is rarely difficult to distinguish haemoptysis from haematemesis but sometimes bleeding from the nose and pharynx may simulate haemoptysis. The amount of blood coughed up can range from large volumes (frank haemoptysis) through blood staining to streaking or flecking of sputum. The most important causes of haemoptysis are pulmonary infarction, bronchial carcinoma, tuberculosis and bronchiectasis. These diseases must always be considered in all patients who cough up blood. Useful diagnostic clues are:

1   Frank haemoptysis usually indicates pulmonary infarction, tuberculosis or bronchiectasis.
2   Haemoptysis preceded by, or associated with, purulent sputum often indicates bronchiectasis, suppurative pneumonia or lung abscess. This kind of 'blood spitting' also occurs in chronic bronchitis.
3   Recurrent blood streaking of sputum must always be regarded as an ominous symptom since the most common cause is bronchial carcinoma.
4   Recurrent haemoptysis over a number of years is more likely to be due to a relatively benign disease, e.g. bronchiectasis.

Table 1.1 Causes of haemoptysis.

Common
   *Pulmonary infarction
   *Bronchial carcinoma
   *Tuberculosis
   *Bronchiectasis
    Suppurative pneumonia
    Lung abscess
    †Acute bronchitis
    †Chronic bronchitis

Uncommon
    Mitral stenosis
    Aspergilloma
    Bronchial adenoma
    Tracheal tumours
    Metastatic pulmonary malignant disease
    Laryngeal tumours
    Connective tissue diseases (SLE)
    Idiopathic pulmonary haemosiderosis
    Goodpasture's syndrome
    Pulmonary arteriovenous malformations
    Blood dyscrasias and anticoagulation
    Hypertension

Others
    Foreign body inhalation
    Accidental chest trauma
    Iatrogenic: bronchoscopy, transbronchial lung biopsy, transthoracic
       lung biopsy

---

*Most important causes.
†Diagnosis assumed only after exclusion of other causes.

Although haemoptysis occurs in simple bronchial infection such as acute bronchitis and infective exacerbations of chronic bronchitis, all patients with this symptom should be considered to have a more serious cause in the first instance. Without this type of approach the diagnosis of diseases such as bronchial carcinoma can be delayed. Chronic bronchitis and bronchial carcinoma often occur together, since both are caused by smoking and, therefore, if a patient with chronic bronchitis has haemoptysis bronchial carcinoma and not chronic bronchitis should be considered to be the cause until it is excluded by the appropriate investigations.

Breathlessness (dyspnoea)

Breathlessness can be said to be present when a patient is aware that breathing involves conscious effort. There are many respiratory causes of breathlessness but the majority can be loosely divided into two main groups:

1 Breathlessness associated with airways obstruction

Airways obstruction increases the work of breathing and is associated with wheeze or stridor.

2 Breathlessness associated with impairment of inflation of the lungs in the absence of airways obstruction (restrictive disease)

Chest wall causes. Neuromuscular — polyneuritis, poliomyelitis and myasthenia gravis. Skeletal — severe chest deformity and ankylosing spondylitis.

Pleural causes. Pleural effusion, pleural fibrosis and pneumothorax.

Pulmonary causes. Any condition which decreases pulmonary compliance (increases the 'stiffness' of the lungs) — fibrosis in its many forms, tumour, especially lymphatic carcinomatosis, pneumonia and oedema.

Hypoxaemia if severe, and especially if sudden in onset, can cause breathlessness by stimulation of receptors in the carotid bodies and aorta. Chemoreceptor stimulation can augment breathlessness in diseases such as acute pulmonary oedema and pulmonary embolism, but in these conditions it is likely that stimulation of J-receptors in the walls of pulmonary capillaries is the main cause of dyspnoea.

Breathlessness is not only a manifestation of almost all bronchopulmonary disease and many of the cardiovascular system, but it is the only respiratory symptom that is a common manifestation of hysteria (hysterical hyperventilation).

IMPORTANT HISTORICAL POINTS

1 Duration.
2 Speed of onset (*see* Table 1.2).

Table 1.2 Rapidity of onset of breathlessness.

Acute onset (minutes/hours)	Subacute onset (days/weeks)	Chronic onset (months/years)
Pneumothorax	Pleural effusion	Chronic bronchitis
Foreign body inhalation	Bronchial asthma	Emphysema
Pulmonary embolism	Exacerbation of chronic bronchitis	Bronchial carcinoma
Bronchial asthma	Pneumonia	Fibrosing alveolitis
Pulmonary oedema	Pulmonary oedema	Lymphatic carcinomatosis
Pneumonia	Bronchial carcinoma	Sarcoidosis
Acute bronchitis	Tuberculosis	Pneumoconiosis
Allergic alveolitis	Lymphatic carcinomatosis	Tuberculosis
Hysterical hyperventilation	Anaemia	Thromboembolic pulmonary hypertension
		Anaemia
		Obesity

3 Association with other symptoms particularly wheeze and chest pain.

4 Relationship to exertion.

5 Spontaneous breathlessness at night — 'paroxysmal nocturnal dyspnoea' — is a very common symptom of cardiac disease, but nocturnal breathlessness is also characteristic of bronchial asthma.

GRADING OF BREATHLESSNESS

Breathlessness, unless it is hysterical, is always made worse by exertion and it is useful clinically to assess the severity of this symptom by relating disability to everyday activity — e.g. breathlessness when walking up hills, on the level or at rest.

Wheeze (and stridor)

Wheeze is frequently associated with breathlessness and is a manifestation of obstructive airways diseases such as asthma and chronic obstructive bronchitis. It is clinically most marked during expiration but only a minority of patients appear to be aware of this. The relationship of wheeze to exertion, changes of temperature and inhalation of bronchial irritants and possible allergens must be determined. It is also important to enquire about nocturnal exacerbations.

Stridor due to partial obstruction of major airways may be mistaken for wheeze, but stridor is always worse on inspiration. In cases where early stridor is suspected it can be accentuated by asking the patient to cough and then to breathe deeply through a widely open mouth.

Pleuritic pain

Pleuritic pain has many causes, but the most common are:
    Infection (simple and tuberculous)
    Pulmonary infarction
    Malignant disease.

It is usually severe and often described as knife-like, and is characteristically made worse by breathing and coughing. Diaphragmatic pleural pain is often referred to the shoulder. The features of pleural pain are so classical that it is rarely mistaken for other types of chest pain except for fractured ribs and epidemic myalgia (Bornholm disease).

Central chest pain of non-pleuritic type may simulate cardiac pain and

is occasionally produced by tumours of the mediastinum, acute mediastinitis and mediastinal emphysema. Central pain, often described as
'burning', is a common symptom of acute inflammation of the trachea
(acute tracheitis).

Examination

General observations

Breathless patients like to sit upright, and those with obstructive airways
disease fix the shoulder girdle to give the accessory muscles more pur-
chase to aid expiration. Pleuritic pain may induce the patient to compress the chest with the hands in an attempt to reduce chest wall movement and always induces shallow rapid breathing. Patients dyspnoeic
because of obstructive airways disease have prolongation of expiration
with clearly audible expiratory wheeze. In contrast, the restrictive
diseases cause rapid breathing without expiratory difficulty. The
presence or absence of cough is readily apparent. Less ill patients should
be observed after exertion (moving in bed, undressing or walking) to
assess the degree of breathlessness. Purse-lip breathing always means
severe and usually irreversible airways disease associated with air
trapping (emphysema).

Cyanosis, if immediately apparent, reflects severe hypoxaemia.
Colour of the tongue in daylight is the best clinical guide of hypoxaemia
of respiratory origin (central cyanosis).

Assessment of higher cerebral functions is of extreme importance in
severely ill patients. Hypoxia of acute onset can induce respiratory distress associated with anxiety. Profound hypoxia can be associated with
confusion, but disordered cerebral function usually means acute carbon
dioxide retention (respiratory acidosis) as well as hypoxia. Drowsiness,
confusion and coma occur in severe hypercapnia and sweating,
twitching and coarse tremor are also characteristic features.

The hands

Careful examination of the hands is vital:

1 *Finger clubbing* (Fig. 1.1). The respiratory causes of finger
clubbing include bronchial carcinoma, intrathoracic suppuration (bronchiectasis, lung abscess and empyema) and fibrosing alveolitis.
2 *Flapping tremor.* Frequently present in uncompensated respiratory acidosis which is much more common than the other cause, liver
failure.

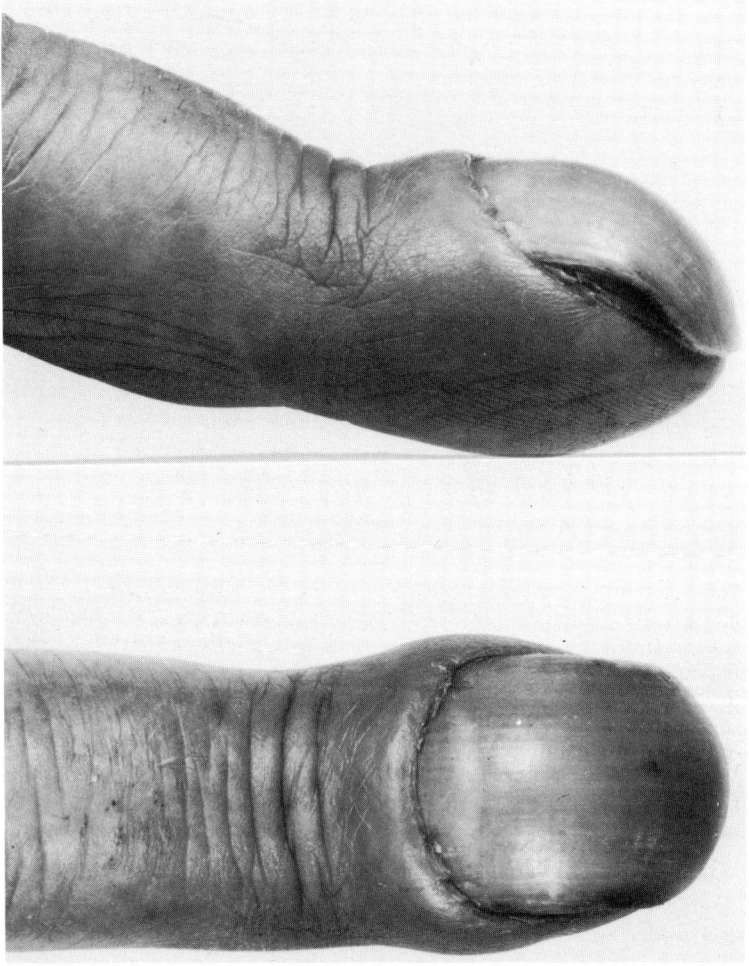

Fig. 1.1   Gross finger clubbing.

3   *Skin temperature of the hands.*   Carbon dioxide retention is associated with warm extremities.

Warm, blue flapping hands are found in acute respiratory acidosis.

The neck

The neck must be carefully examined systematically. Engorgement of neck veins can be due to increased intrathoracic pressure during expira-

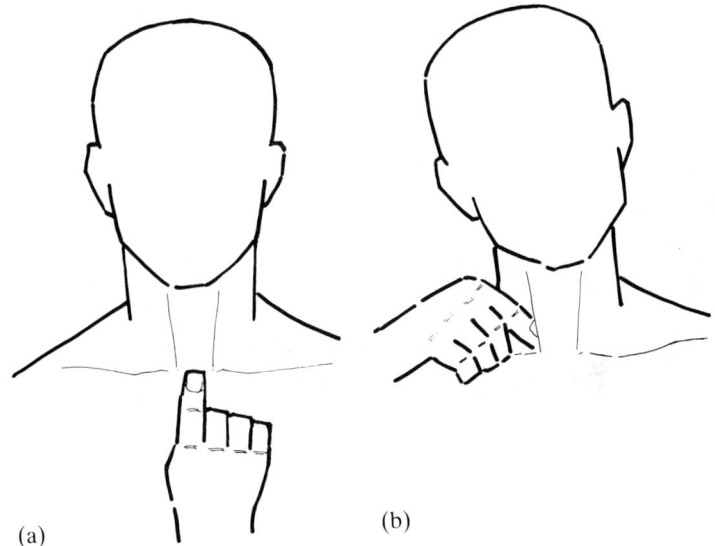

(a) (b)

Fig. 1.2 (a) Single-finger palpation of the neck above the suprasternal notch to determine the position of the trachea. (b) Palpation of the scalene area of the neck of enlargement of lymph glands. Patient's head tilted to the side being examined in order to relax the sternomastoid muscle.

tion, right ventricular failure or superior vena caval obstruction. Palpation will determine the position of the trachea (Fig. 1.2a) and enlargement of supraclavicular nodes (Fig. 1.2b). Subcutaneous emphysema is usually easily detectable in the neck by palpation.

The eyes

Conjunctival oedema is present in many patients with respiratory failure and cor pulmonale. Horner's syndrome may indicate an apical bronchial carcinoma. Examination of the fundi will reveal engorgement of retinal veins and occasionally papilloedema in patients with type II respiratory failure, and a thorough search for choroidal tubercles must be made in patients thought to have miliary tuberculosis.

The precordium

Conditions causing pulmonary hypertension will result in right ventricular hypertrophy which can be detected clinically by palpating with the flat of the hand a left parasternal impulse. On auscultation the pulmonary component of the second heart sound may be accentuated and there may be a third heart sound audible. In the presence of emphysema it is often not possible to palpate a right ventricular pulsation or hear heart sounds clearly because of overinflated lung between the heart and the anterior chest wall.

Dependent oedema may be an early feature of cor pulmonale (p. 34) and later becomes associated with hepatomegaly and elevation of the jugular venous pressure.

The upper respiratory tract

Examination of the nose, mouth, pharynx and larynx, in selected cases, is of course essential. Nasal mucosal swelling and polyp formation is common in patients with allergic disorders.

The chest

There is a tendency for the inexperienced to denigrate the value of clinical examination of the chest and place too much emphasis on radiological findings. Precise diagnosis, however, depends upon the proper interpretation of abnormal clinical findings, together with information provided by the chest X-rays. The routine examination of the chest by inspection, palpation, percussion and auscultation is often performed well by inexperienced clinicians, but lack of appreciation of the significance of abnormal findings may lead to misinterpretation. The relevance of each abnormality must be considered as it is detected (e.g. diminished expansion on inspection) so that abnormal signs subsequently elicited (e.g. dull percussion note) should be anticipated in order to allow appreciation of the significance of auscultatory findings (e.g. absent breath sounds: diagnosis — pleural effusion or collapse). Such an examination technique is much more rewarding than trying to assess the relevance of a host of abnormalities at the end of physical examination.

INSPECTION

The rate and depth of breathing as well as the presence of expiratory wheeze, inspiratory stridor and obvious pain associated with breathing must be noted.

CHEST SHAPE ABNORMALITIES

The most important abnormalities of chest configuration are:

Increase in anteroposterior diameter (barrel chest)

This usually reflects long-standing chronic obstructive airways disease but can be due to air trapping in severe asthma. Genuine increase in AP diameter is always associated with decreased chest expansion and accompanied by use of the accessory muscles (sternomastoids, scaleni and trapezii) which lift the thorax on inspiration but do not necessarily increase expansion. Thus chest movement and expansion are precise terms and are not interchangeable.

Indrawing of intercostal spaces is evidence of marked airways obstruction and is often seen in patients with barrel chest deformity.

Pectus carinatum ('pigeon' chest; Fig 1.3a)

Chronic inflation of the lungs in children, almost always due to asthma, causes the characteristic forward bowing of the sternum and indrawing of the lower lateral ribs due to muscular pull of the insertions of the diaphragm (Harrison's sulci).

Thoracic kyphoscoliosis

This is not due to respiratory disease but often causes respiratory problems in adult life because of the ventilation–perfusion imbalance it can produce. Scoliosis produces more respiratory embarrassment than kyphosis.

Pectus excavatum ('funnel' chest; Fig. 1.3b)

This congenital depression of the lower sternum is often cosmetically embarrassing but rarely causes respiratory disease.

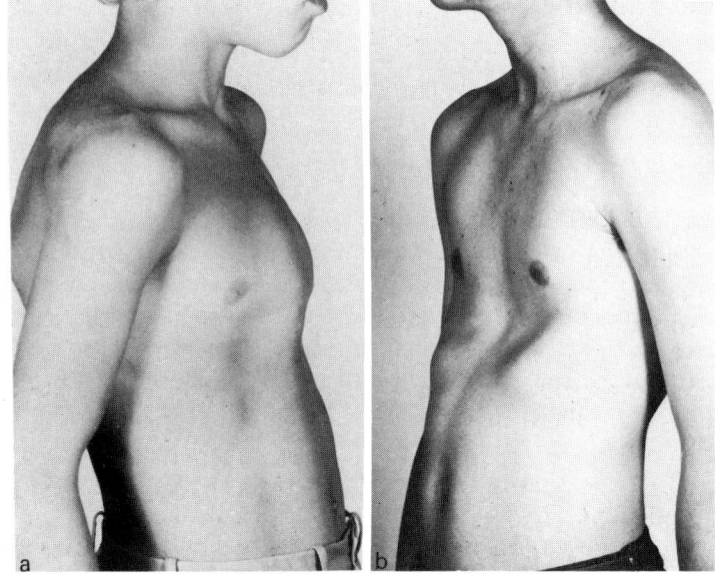

Fig. 1.3 (a) Pectus carinatum ('pigeon' chest). (b) Pectus excavatum ('funnel' chest).

Deformities due to accidental trauma and thoracic operations

Most deformities due to uncorrected chest trauma and thoracoplasty operations (rarely performed today) can lead to ventilation-perfusion imbalance.

Lesions of chest wall not associated with deformity. Scars, bruising, eruptions, nodules, swelling, dilated veins, etc. can all be evidence of intrathoracic pathology.

Decreased expansion in absence of chest deformity. Asymmetrical expansion may be apparent on inspection in some cases of gross pleural and pulmonary pathology.

PALPATION

Routine palpation of the chest wall in the search for nodules, localized tenderness, breast lesions and enlarged axillary lymph nodes should precede assessment of chest expansion.

CHEST EXPANSION

Common abnormalities of chest expansion are given in Table 1.3. In the absence of chest deformity, the important abnormalities are:

Bilateral diminution of expansion

This is a feature of:

1 All patients with pleuritic pain — pain limits inspiratory effort — chest shape frequently normal — common.
2 Hyperinflation of lungs causing fixation of ribs in the inspiratory position — chest shape abnormal (barrel chest) — common.
3 Bilateral pulmonary diseases causing gross restriction of expansion — e.g. fibrosing alveolitis, lymphatic carcinomatosis — uncommon.
4 Bilateral pleural abnormalities causing restrictive defect — e.g. bilateral pleural effusions and fibrosis — uncommon.
5 Musculoskeletal diseases — causing restriction of chest expansion

Table 1.3 Some causes of decreased chest expansion.

Bilateral	Unilateral
Lung hyperinflation Emphysema Asthma	*Lung hyperinflation* Obstructive emphysema (rare)
Restrictive lung diseases Fibrosing alveolitis Allergic alveolitis Lymphatic carcinomatosis Sarcoidosis	*Pulmonary disorders* Collapse Consolidation Localized fibrosis Large peripheral tumour
Pleural diseases Pleuritic pain Bilateral effusions Bilateral fibrosis (rare)	*Pleural diseases* Pneumothorax Pleural effusion Empyema Pleural fibrosis Pleural tumour (rare)
Musculoskeletal disorders Myasthenia gravis Polyneuropathies Ankylosing spondylitis Kyphosis	*Musculoskeletal disorders* Scoliosis

— e.g. myasthenia gravis, polyneuropathies or ankylosing spondylitis — uncommon.

Unilateral diminution of chest expansion

This is an important and common abnormal finding. The side of decreased chest expansion can always be regarded as the abnormal side. The commonest causes are:

1 Pleural — effusion, fibrosis, and pneumothorax.
2 Pulmonary — collapse, consolidation, localized fibrosis and rarely large peripheral tumour.

PERCUSSION

The percussion note may be normal, dull or hyper-resonant. It is easier to be confident about the presence of dullness than hyper-resonance.

Bilateral hyper-resonance is present in emphysema together with other signs of pulmonary hyperinflation such as bilaterally decreased expansion, use of accessory muscles, decreased cardiac dullness and poor air entry. In the absence of chest distension a 'hyper-resonant' percussion note may simply reflect a thin chest wall.

Unilateral hyper-resonant percussion note can be elicited over pneumothorax, large bullae and thin-walled pulmonary cysts or abscesses.

A hyper-resonant or tympanitic note is elicited over an air-containing viscus (stomach or colon), and this is therefore quite often found over the left lower thorax. It may be a sign of paralysis of the left hemidiaphragm.

Dull percussion note

Impairment of the percussion note is produced by any pulmonary lesion which decreases alveolar aeration (collapse, consolidation, gross localized fibrosis and, rarely, large peripheral tumour masses) or any process which causes increased density of the pleura (effusion, fibrosis or tumour). Elevation of the right hemidiaphragm may simulate right-sided pleural disease or pathology in the right lower lobe. Whenever impairment of percussion note is elicited the side of the dull percussion note is usually the abnormal one.

The dullest percussion note is found over a large pleural effusion (stony dullness). Cardiac dullness is decreased in emphysema when aerated lung is interposed between the heart and the anterior chest wall. Percussion of liver dullness is useful to assess the level of the right hemidiaphragm, but tidal percussion of diaphragm movement is rarely of clinical value.

AUSCULTATION

Special attention should be paid to the detection of:

1 Changes of normal breath sounds
    (a) Decreased intensity
    (b) Absent breath sounds
    (c) Prolongation of expiratory phase.
2 Grossly abnormal breath sounds
    (a) Bronchial breath sounds.
3 Additional noises (added or adventitious sounds)
    (a) Rhonchi
    (b) Crepitations (crackles)
    (c) Pleural friction rub
    (d) Air in abnormal sites.
4 Alteration of voice sounds
    (a) Decreased vocal resonance
    (b) Increased vocal resonance.

Changes of normal breath sounds

Decreased intensity of normal breath sounds is an extremely important abnormal finding, the significance of which is frequently overlooked. Bilateral uniform diminution of breath sounds is common in emphysema, but may be an apparent abnormality in patients with thick chest walls. Localized diminution, or absence of breath sounds, indicates gross pathology. The most common causes are:

(a) Obstruction (partial or complete) of a major bronchus — usually by bronchial carcinoma.
(b) Pleural effusion.
(c) Pneumothorax.

Less common causes are large peripheral lung tumour, pleural tumour and pleural fibrosis.

Grossly abnormal breath sounds

Bronchial breathing will be heard when there is a patent bronchus and an uniform conducting medium between it and the chest wall. Classically it is associated with pneumonic consolidation and, less commonly, dense localized pulmonary fibrosis. It is extremely uncommon to hear bronchial breathing in a patient with bronchial obstruction except in some cases of upper lobe collapse when bronchial-like breath sounds are transmitted from the displaced trachea. Hence it is rare to hear bronchial breathing in bronchial carcinoma. Bronchial breath sounds are sometimes audible over the upper level of a pleural effusion, but this is a rare finding and the mechanism is difficult to explain.

The terms 'aegophony' and 'amphoric bronchial breath sounds' are sometimes used to describe bronchial breathing supposed to be characteristic of different pathologies.

Additional noises (added or adventitious sounds)

Rhonchi are mainly expiratory noises caused by bronchial narrowing often associated with prolongation of expiration. The pitch of the rhonchi relates to the calibre of the narrowed airways. High-pitched rhonchi are most often heard in asthma. Low-pitched rhonchi, which may also be audible on inspiration, are often due to secretions in the large bronchi and clear with coughing.

In some patients with partial obstruction of a large bronchus by tumour or foreign body, a rhonchus not altered by coughing may be audible in one site ('fixed rhonchus') in the absence of rhonchi elsewhere.

Crepitations or crackles are mainly inspiratory noises and are caused by secretions in the alveoli, bronchioles and bronchi, with the important exception of fibrosing alveolitis. Crepitations can be fine, medium and coarse. In general, fine and medium crepitations are caused by pathologies in the alveoli, bronchioles and small bronchi, e.g. pneumonia and pulmonary oedema, and coarse crepitations are due to secretions in larger bronchi, e.g. bronchiectasis. However, allergic and fibrosing alveolitis are characteristically associated with loud end-inspiratory crepitations.

Subcutaneous emphysema causes superficial crackling noises which can be mistaken for genuine crepitations, as can a hairy chest, especially if the diaphragm of the stethoscope is used.

Pleural friction rub. This creaking noise is loudest at the end of inspiration and the beginning of expiration. Friction rubs may not be audible during quiet breathing or in patients with pleuritic pain until adequate analgesia allows deep breaths to be taken. In general, the commonest causes of pleural friction also cause pleuritic pain — pneumonia, pulmonary infarction and tuberculosis. Pleural pain is usually less severe in malignant disease. Loud and sometimes palpable pleural friction, often without pain, is found in connective tissue diseases, e.g. rheumatoid disease. Pleural friction may be confused with low-pitched rhonchi (usually clear or alter with coughing) and a scapular creak (an uncommon skeletal noise of no clinical significance).

Abnormal noises due to air in abnormal sites. A systolic click may be heard in pneumothorax. In mediastinal emphysema cardiac crunching noises may be heard, which can be mistaken for pericardial friction.

Voice sounds (vocal resonance)

Bronchial breathing can be confirmed by the presence of increased vocal resonance to the point of 'whispering pectoriloquy'. Decreased vocal resonance is found over collapse and pleural effusion. It is useful, therefore, to listen to voice noises in all patients in whom a dull percussion note has been elicited.

Investigations

Radiological examination

X-ray examination of the chest is of paramount importance in the investigation of most patients with respiratory disease. Even though an obvious lesion may be immediately visible the systematic examination of all X-rays must include:

1 Soft-tissue shadows including any artefacts due to clothing, dressings on the chest wall, etc.
2 The bony structures.
3 The contours and positions of the hemidiaphragms.
4 The mediastinal structures.
5 The lung fields, with particular reference to the positions of the fissures when visible.

It must be appreciated that the site of a pulmonary lesion cannot be

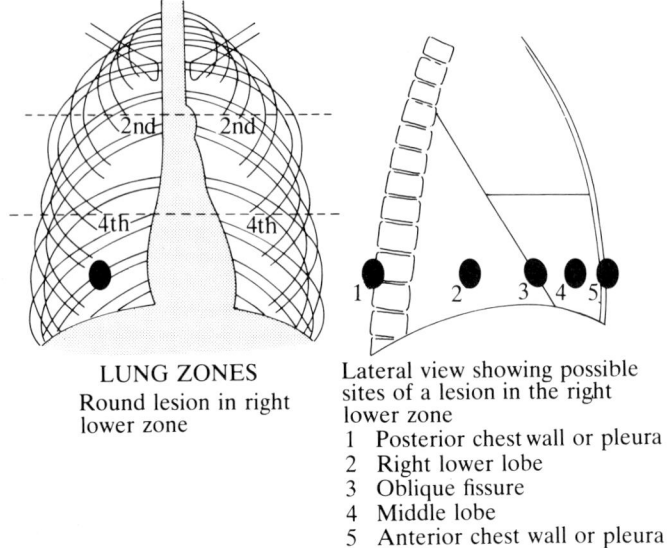

LUNG ZONES
Round lesion in right
lower zone

Lateral view showing possible
sites of a lesion in the right
lower zone
1 Posterior chest wall or pleura
2 Right lower lobe
3 Oblique fissure
4 Middle lobe
5 Anterior chest wall or pleura

Fig. 1.4

accurately determined by examination of a PA or AP X-ray. A lateral
view is required to localize abnormalities within lobes or segments. For
descriptive purposes the straight X-ray is arbitrarily divided into three
zones — upper, mid and lower — separated by horizontal lines
between the anterior ends of the second and fourth ribs (Fig. 1.4). Thus
an abnormality can confidently be stated to be in the right lower zone,
but a lateral film has to be examined to determine the anatomical site of
the lesion.

Chest X-rays frequently show abnormalities but rarely give an
absolute diagnosis (except in the case of pneumothorax) since
pulmonary and pleural lesions of different pathologies produce similar
appearances. For example, a pleural effusion is easily detected because
of its characteristic shape (p. 167), but the pathological cause of the
effusion is only rarely apparent. Pulmonary shadows, whether single or
multiple, also only indicate abnormality since rarely are the X-ray
changes absolutely diagnostic. All X-ray abnormalities if pulmonary
and/or pleural should initially at least be considered to be due to four
common disease categories: (1) simple infections; (2) tuberculosis; (3)
tumour; (4) disorders secondary to cardiovascular disease — pulmonary
infarction and pulmonary oedema. When these common conditions,

which are responsible for the vast majority of X-ray abnormalities, have been considered and the diagnosis is still not readily apparent the rarer causes of pulmonary and pleural lesions should be contemplated. These include: sarcoidosis, industrial lung diseases, connective tissue disorders, fibrosing alveolitis, allergic alveolitis, fungal infections, etc.

SIMPLE INFLAMMATORY LESIONS

Pneumonic consolidation causes confluent shadowing within a segment, lobe or lung and is not associated with alteration of the position of lung fissures. Bronchopneumonia (or lobular pneumonia) causes patchy lobular shadows which may or may not be confined to one lobe, and the diagnosis from X-ray alone can be difficult since other pathological processes often cause similar X-ray abnormalities.

TUBERCULOSIS

Tuberculosis has a predilection for the upper lobes, especially the apices, and is commonly bilateral. Cavitation within an area of pulmonary shadowing in an upper lobe should always raise the possibility of TB. However, TB is by no means always a disease of the apices. Tuberculous bronchopneumonia is indistinguishable radiographically from simple bacterial pneumonia. Miliary tuberculosis has an almost characteristic appearance because of the 'miliary shadowing', with lesions of 1–2 mm diameter. The individual X-ray shadows, however, can be much larger (up to 10 mm), and similar lesions can be produced by a variety of other diseases, notably simple bacterial infection, malignant disease, sarcoidosis and pneumoconiosis.

TUMOURS

Bronchial carcinoma frequently presents radiographically as collapse/ consolidation, and hence displacement of fissures indicating shrinkage of pulmonary tissue should always suggest bronchial obstruction due to carcinoma. Unilateral hilar prominence is a frequent finding. Peripheral tumours are usually obvious, unless very small, but often the radiographic features simulate tuberculosis or a simple inflammatory lesion. Multiple pulmonary tumour deposits when large can give the 'cannonball' picture, but by no means always, and multiple small tumour metastases can mimic the many conditions associated with diffuse pulmonary mottling — bronchopneumonia, miliary tuberculosis, sarcoidosis, pneumoconiosis, allergic and fibrosing alveolitis, etc. Great care must be taken in the examination of skeletal structures since bone erosion is rarely caused by non-malignant diseases.

PLEUROPULMONARY DISORDERS SECONDARY TO CARDIOVASCULAR DISEASE

Pulmonary oedema and pulmonary infarction are very common causes of X-ray abnormality, but are often overlooked, even by experienced clinicians, in the differential diagnosis of pulmonary shadowing and pleural effusion. Pulmonary oedema may cause unilateral X-ray abnormality. It is not the sole cause of septal lines (Kerley's B lines, Fig. 1.5) which are also seen in lymphatic carcinomatosis and occasionally in pneumoconiosis. The radiographic abnormalities of pulmonary infarction are predominantly in the lower zones and frequently associated with pleural opacities and linear shadows. However, pulmonary infarction is misdiagnosed as pneumonia on frequent occasions. The differential diagnosis of bilateral lower zone shadowing must always include pulmonary infarction.

Tomography

Tomography, which provides films of sections of the intrathoracic

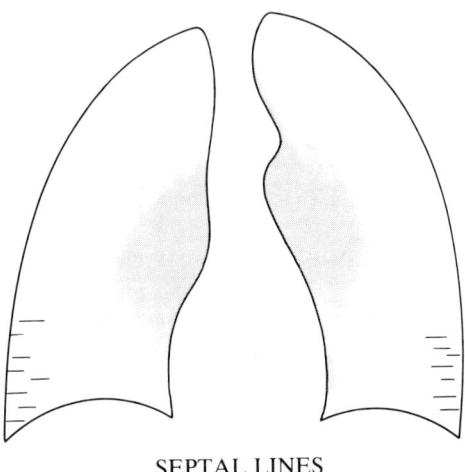

SEPTAL LINES

Fig. 1.5 Diagrammatic representation of X-ray showing septal lines (Kerley's B lines).

structures 'in focus' at different levels, can be helpful in cases where plain radiography fails to demonstrate lesions clearly. The main indications for tomography are:

Confirmation or exclusion of a cavity within an abnormality visible on the plain X-ray. Cavitation is most frequently due to lung abscess or suppurative pneumonia, tuberculosis and necrosis within a tumour mass. An irregular and thick-walled cavity usually indicates necrosis within a tumour mass. Tomography may also reveal a fungus ball within a cavity (p. 125).

Demonstration of calcification within solid lesions. The presence of calcification suggests that the lesion is a tuberculoma or simple tumour, but calcification does not exclude a diagnosis of carcinoma.

Investigation of a prominent hilar shadow.   Tomography can differentiate between enlargement of hilar glands and prominence of hilar vessels and hence can be of considerable value in the investigation of patients with bronchial carcinoma who have suspected hilar glandular involvement.

Investigation of mediastinal masses.   The extent of mediastinal masses is often difficult to define with plain radiography and when this is the case tomography is sometimes useful, but seldom gives as much information as CT scanning (*see below*).

To aid diagnosis by providing evidence not visible on the plain X-rays. In the investigation of the solitary pulmonary shadow tomography may show multiple line shadows radiating from a solid lesion, which strongly suggests a diagnosis of carcinoma, or small satellite lesions, which are more often seen in tuberculosis than carcinoma.

Investigation of tracheal or main bronchus narrowing.   Tomography is much more helpful than plain radiology in the localization of the site of narrowing of a major bronchus but should not be used as an alternative to bronchoscopy.

In general AP tomograms are most useful but lateral and AP tomography together may be necessary in the investigation of hilar lesions.

COMPUTERIZED AXIAL TOMOGRAPHY (CT)

This investigation is not available in all hospitals because of the cost of scanners. CT is based on the density of the body tissues to X-rays, and hence the cross-sectional views produced by CT scanners are as easily understood as conventional X-rays. The cross-sectional nature of CT avoids superimposition of structures, and it is a sensitive technique which can show fine structures and small changes in tissue density representing pathology which may not be visible on the conventional X-ray.

CT is particularly useful in the investigation of mediastinal abnormalities (p. 299) and in bronchopulmonary disease such as bronchial carcinoma and secondary pulmonary metastatic disease (p. 146). It is of definite benefit in the staging of patients with malignant disease. Also, it has been used in the diagnosis of emphysema (p. 44) and clearly defines pleural and chest wall lesions. Its true value in the investigation of some other thoracic disorders has yet to be clearly established.

Bronchography

Bronchography is best performed under general anaesthesia at the same time as bronchoscopy in the investigation of bronchiectasis. The most common indication for this combined procedure is haemoptysis. Bronchoscopy is performed first to exclude a diagnosis of carcinoma, and also to remove by suction excess bronchial secretions, which if present usually make bronchography technically imperfect.

'Selective bronchography' can be performed by injecting the radio-opaque contrast medium into lobar or segmental bronchi using a fibre-optic bronchoscope and local anaesthesia.

Screening (fluoroscopy) and barium swallow

These are routine investigations of bronchial carcinoma in order to detect phrenic nerve paralysis (paradoxical movement of the hemidiaphragm on sniffing), and tumour deposits in the mediastinum causing indentation and displacement of the barium-outlined oesophagus. Screening is also used in the localization of pulmonary lesions for the purposes of transbronchial and percutaneous biopsy procedures.

Pulmonary angiography

Angiography is essential in the management of massive pulmonary embolism if surgical treatment is contemplated, and also in the investigation of pulmonary hypertension.

Radioisotope lung scanning

Perfusion lung scans are of undoubted value in pulmonary thromboembolic disease, and ventilation/perfusion scanning may improve diagnostic accuracy and provide useful information in a wide variety of bronchopulmonary disorders.

Gallium-67 scans. Gallium-67 is taken up by 'inflammatory' cells. Normal lungs have virtually no uptake of this isotope, but in infections and the diffuse lung diseases (e.g. fibrosing alveolitis and pulmonary sarcoidosis) there is increased uptake. The increase in fibrosing alveolitis correlates well with cellular histology and in sarcoidosis reflects the degree of disease activity. The role of gallium-67 scanning in diseases associated with an alveolitis has yet to be fully defined.

Using first-pass radionuclide imaging, right ventricular function can be assessed by measurement of 'right ventricular ejection fraction'. This could be of value in following the progress of patients with right ventricular problems secondary to lung disease, e.g. hypoxic cor pulmonale caused by chronic bronchitis.

Pulmonary function tests

Measurement of function of the bronchi and lungs is very important in the investigation of many bronchopulmonary disorders. There are few patients who cannot be adequately investigated using readily available techniques, and referral to a fully equipped respiratory physiology laboratory should rarely be necessary providing correct interpretation is made of the results of simple tests. The basic measurements on which most diagnostic and therapeutic decisions can be made are:

1 Ventilatory function tests.
2 Lung volume measurements.
3 Transfer factor (diffusing capacity).
4 Arterial blood gas analysis.
5 Exercise tests.

VENTILATORY FUNCTION TESTS

For routine clinical purposes estimates of resistance to air flow in the tracheobronchial system can be made by simple spirometry. The volume of gas expired by maximal effort after a full inspiration is the forced vital capacity (FVC). By using one of the many simple instruments available the volume of air expelled in the first second of the forced expiratory manoeuvre — forced expiratory volume in one second (FEV_1) — can also be readily measured. An FEV_1/FVC ratio of 75–80% indicates normal airways function (Fig. 1.6a). A ratio of less than 70% is evidence of expiratory air flow obstruction (Fig. 1.6b). In restrictive disorders the FVC is reduced but the FEV_1 is normal. The FEV_1/FVC ratio is therefore over 80%, and in extreme cases the FEV_1 and the FVC are the same.

Peak expiratory flow (PEF) is the peak flow at the beginning of an expiration delivered with maximal force from a fully inflated chest. This closely correlates with the FEV_1, and provides a readily available measurement of airways function. Cheap gauges are in use which allow selected patients to record PEF regularly, at least twice daily. This often provides valuable diagnostic information (differentiating between chronic asthma and chronic bronchitis, confirming occupational asthma, etc.), and self-monitoring of PEF also allows asthmatic patients to make adjustments to their treatment on objective recordings rather than on symptoms. The PEF is of no value in the assessment of restrictive pulmonary diseases (p. 6).

LUNG VOLUMES (Fig. 1.7)

Estimation of total lung capacity (TLC), vital capacity (VC), residual volume (RV) and the other subdivisions of TLC are particularly helpful in the diagnosis of restrictive disorders. The RV is the air left in the lungs after full expiration. It is increased, together with the TLC (RV + VC), in diseases associated with lung hyperinflation, notably emphysema, although the VC itself is frequently reduced, though not as much as the FEV_1. The TLC and all its subdivisions are below normal predicted values in restrictive diseases, e.g. fibrosing alveolitis. It follows that measurement of VC alone is not very helpful. Recording of 'relaxed' VC (total amount of air exhaled after full inspiration but not during a forced expiratory manoeuvre) is often more useful than the FVC in obstructive airways disease since forced expiration often increases the degree of air trapping.

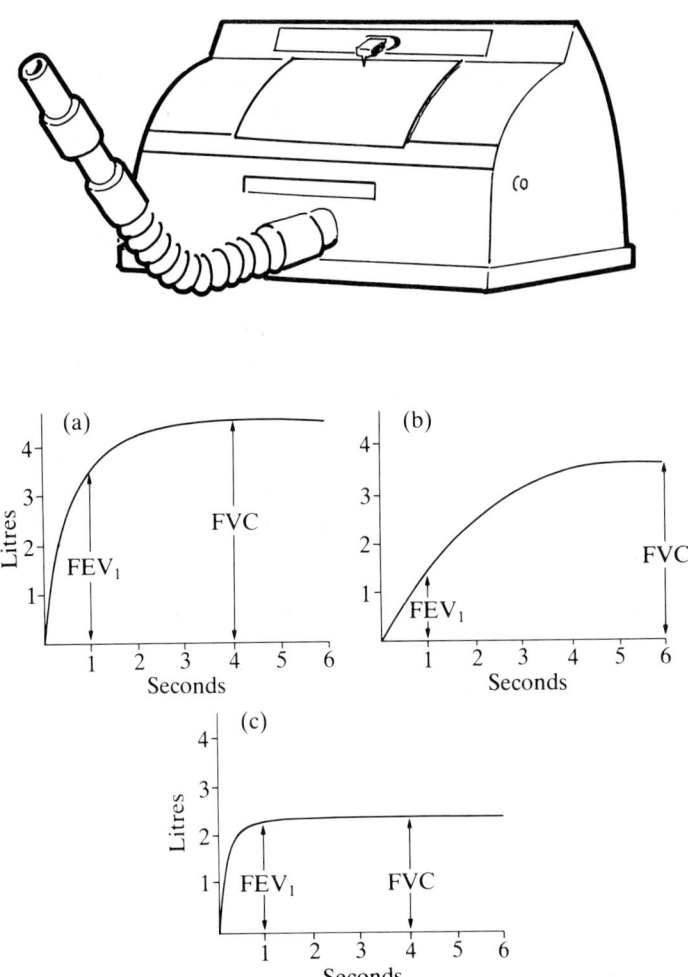

Fig. 1.6 Spirometry (Vitalograph) tracings showing the relationship of FEV_1 to FVC. (a) Normal. (b) Airways obstruction. (c) Restrictive defect.

FLOW–VOLUME LOOP

In this test the rates at which air flows out of and into the lungs during forced maximum expiration and inspiration are measured and plotted against volume on some form of X–Y recorder (Fig. 1.8) Flow rates are decreased with airways collapse and the expiratory limb is scooped out

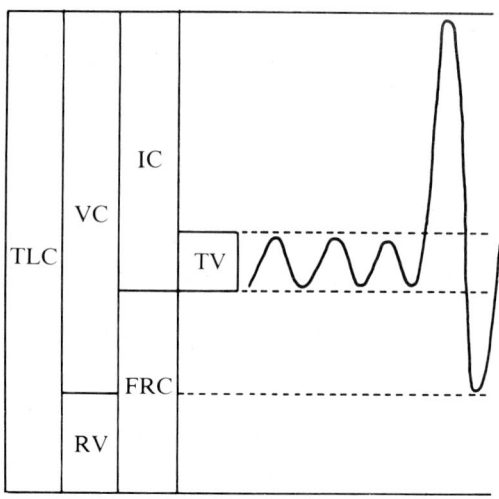

Fig. 1.7 Lung volumes. TLC, total lung capacity; VC, Vital capacity; RV, residual volume; IC, inspiratory capacity; FRC, functional residual capacity; TV, tidal volume.

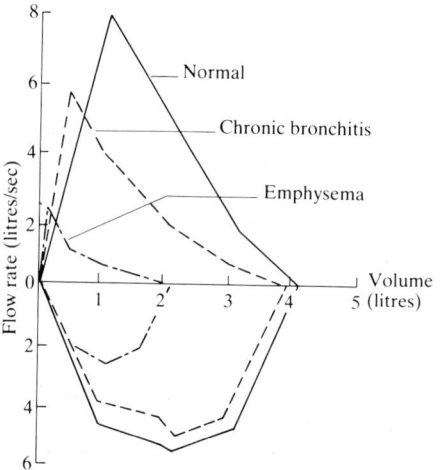

Fig. 1.8 Flow–volume loops. Normal, chronic bronchitis, and emphysema.

compared with the almost straight line seen in health. Flow–volume loops can be of value in assessing upper airways obstruction, e.g. tracheal tumour or stenosis.

TRANSFER FACTOR (DIFFUSING CAPACITY)

Measurement of transfer factor for carbon monoxide provides a useful index of severity of restrictive lung diseases such as fibrosing alveolitis. However, transfer factor as presently estimated does not simply reflect the permeability of the membrane separating alveolar gas from pulmonary capillary blood, but is also intimately dependent upon alveolar ventilation and perfusion. Thus abnormalities of transfer factor will be found in all diseases in which there is ventilation/perfusion imbalance. Transfer factor measurements are, therefore, of greatest value in patients with restrictive lung diseases in whom there is no co-existent airways or vascular disorder.

ARTERIAL BLOOD GAS ANALYSIS

Measurements of arterial blood tensions of oxygen and carbon dioxide together with pH or hydrogen ion concentration are routine investigations of most respiratory disorders and are essential in the management of diseases such as asthma and chronic bronchitis. Most patients with restrictive disorders will be found to have hypoxaemia either at rest or on exercise but the carbon dioxide tension will be normal or low reflecting alveolar hyperventilation (type I respiratory failure). In these patients the pH or hydrogen ion concentration may show a respiratory alkalosis. Alveolar hypoventilation is reflected by carbon dioxide retention and respiratory acidosis (type II respiratory failure).

EXERCISE TESTS

Twelve-minute walking test.   The distance a breathless patient is able to walk at this own pace during a set time such as 12 or 6 minutes provides a good and reproducible estimate of the degree of exercise limitation caused by bronchopulmonary disease. Repeat tests are a useful way of assessing response to treatment, e.g. corticosteroids in chronic obstructive airways disease.

Formal progressive exercise testing.   The tests most often used in the investigation of breathless patients in whom the diagnosis is in doubt involve measurements made during incremental exercise on a cycle ergometer or treadmill. Information is derived from recordings of tidal volume, respiratory rate, expiratory flow patterns, oxygen uptake, carbon dioxide output, heart rate, electrocardiographic changes and arterial oxygen saturation measured by ear oximetry. These tests give an index of maximum exercise capacity and also help to determine whether breathlessness is due to cardiovascular, respiratory or psychogenic problems.

Diagnostic procedures

Bronchoscopy

Visualization of the trachea and bronchi is of paramount importance in the investigation of suspected bronchial carcinoma. The development of the fibreoptic bronchoscope has extended the use of bronchoscopy, since this instrument allows biopsy and brushings to be taken from peripheral lesions (solid and diffuse) and also has extended the use of bronchoalveolar lavage (*see below*).

DIAGNOSTIC BRONCHOSCOPY

A rigid or fibreoptic instrument can be used. (Occasionally the fibre-optic instrument can be passed through the rigid bronchoscope, but this entails the risk of damaging the expensive fibreoscope.) Normally bronchoscopy using the rigid instrument is performed under general anaesthesia with Venturi ventilation, and fibreoptic bronchoscopy is performed with local anaesthesia, the instrument usually being introduced nasally. The rigid bronchoscope allows efficient suction of blood and mucus and the biopsy forceps take a large fragment of tissue which is usually appreciated by the pathologist, especially when tumours are necrotic. The fibreoptic instrument gives improved access to the upper lobar and all segmental bronchi so that forceps, bronchial brush or lavage material can be obtained more easily from peripheral lesions. Extrabronchial tumours lying adjacent to central bronchi or malignant involvement of subcarinal nodes can be sampled by transbronchial needle aspiration biopsy using either instrument.

THERAPEUTIC BRONCHOSCOPY

Removal of sections by suction is essential in patients unable to cough efficiently (respiratory failure due to chronic obstructive airways disease or neurological disorders). In general, aspiration by suction is much more efficient with the rigid instrument, but the fibreoscope is of great value in a patient with an endotracheal tube or tracheostomy.

BRONCHOALVEOLAR LAVAGE (BAL)

Bronchoalveolar lavage via the fibreoptic bronchoscope was developed in the early 1970s as an extension of earlier lung lavage techniques using balloon-tipped catheters via the rigid bronchoscope. The technique is performed by wedging the tip of the bronchoscope into a subsegmental bronchus and instilling warmed saline in 20–50 ml aliquots followed by immediate aspiration under gentle (less than 100 mmHg) suction. Generally, a total lavage volume of between 100 and 300 ml is used. From normal lungs approximately 65–70% of the instilled fluid is recovered, but in patients with severe airflow obstruction (e.g. emphysema) the recoverable volume diminishes markedly.

BAL fluid samples cells and organisms of the bronchoalveolar regions and also the proteins and other constituents of the bronchoalveolar lining fluids. It can, therefore, be used in diagnosis, in the assessment of patients with interstitial lung diseases, and in the research into the patho-genetic processes of a wide spectrum of pulmonary disorders.

As a diagnostic tool BAL has proved to be useful in the investigation of pulmonary tumours and infections. Cytological examination of the cells recovered may enable the diagnosis of peripheral lung tumours or disseminated secondary malignancy, while microbiological examination can achieve a rapid diagnosis of tuberculosis in patients unable to produce sputum, and the identification of organisms responsible for 'opportunistic' infections in immunosuppressed patients.

In patients with interstitial lung diseases the proportions of the various cell types recovered at BAL may differ from normal. In fibrosing alveolitis there are increases in neutrophils and eosinophils, while in sarcoidosis and extrinsic allergic alveolitis increases in lymphocytes are found. The initial optimistic prognostic implication based upon the various proportions of cells found in the different inter-stitial lung diseases have not been completely substantiated. However, monoclonal antibody staining of the lymphocytes has revealed further patterns within the disease groups, e.g. predominance of helper/inducer T-cells in sarcoidosis. Whether such developments will assist the clini-cian is debatable.

Other biopsy techniques

Pleural biopsy performed at the time of aspiration of a pleural effusion is a simple and safe technique which greatly increases the likelihood of establishing a positive diagnosis, especially in tuberculous and malignant effusions. Biopsy of pleural lesions can also be performed under vision (thoracoscopy).

Lymph node aspiration and biopsy

Biopsy or fine-needle aspiration of enlarged cervical glands (especially scalene nodes) should be performed whenever they are palpable and a diagnosis has not been established. Needle aspiration of glands is a simple procedure, and cytological examination of the tissue/fluid obtained can avoid a formal gland biopsy in many cases. Mediastinal glands around the trachea and main bronchi are accessible to mediastinoscopy (p. 148). Needle aspirates from subcarinal glands can be taken via the bronchoscope.

Percutaneous lung biopsy

In selected cases with the aid of X-ray screening peripheral lung lesions can be aspirated or biopsied directly through the chest wall using a long fine needle.

Cytology

Examination for malignant cells of pleural liquid, sputum, bronchial aspirates or brushings and gland or tumour aspirates can be invaluable in the diagnosis of malignant disorders.

Further reading

Clark T.J.H. (1981) *Clinical Investigation of Respiratory Disease.* London: Chapman & Hall Ltd.
Cotes J.E. (1979) *Lung Function: Assessment and Application in Medicine,* 4th Edition. Oxford: Blackwell Scientific Publications.
Forgacs P. (1978) *Lung Sounds.* London: Baillière Tindall.
Lehrer S. (1984) *Understanding Lung Sounds.* Philadelphia: W. B. Saunders.
Macleod J. (1986) *Clinical Examination,* 7th Edition. Edinburgh: Churchill Livingstone.
Naidich D.P., Zerhouni E.A. & Siegelman S.S. (1984) *Computed Tomography of the Thorax.* New York: Raven Press.

Chapter 2
Chronic bronchitis

General considerations

Daily cough productive of sputum for at least three consecutive months in the year, for at least two consecutive years, is the accepted definition of chronic bronchitis. This definition, however, bears little relation to the disease in its advanced form which causes around 30 000 deaths annually in the United Kingdom, and is responsible for disability in about one million patients. The major cause of chronic bronchitis is cigarette smoking, but bronchial irritation from certain dusty occupations, air pollution and climatic conditions are contributing factors. It is a disease of the middle-aged and elderly and is more common in males than females. Hypersecretion of bronchial mucus and airways obstruction are fundamental abnormalities in chronic bronchitis.

Fundamental points of diagnosis

Diagnosis is predominantly based on the history. It is useful to categorize patients into two main groups depending on the degree of airways obstruction present:

Chronic bronchitis with little or no obstructive airways disease

Symptoms of cough and sputum without wheeze and breathlessness. 'Simple chronic bronchitis' and 'chronic recurrent mucopurulent bronchitis' are terms used to describe this type of disease which is predominantly due to mucous gland hypertrophy and hypersecretion with or without episodes of bronchial infection.

Chronic bronchitis associated with obstructive airways disease

'Chronic obstructive bronchitis'. Cough productive of sputum but also chronic breathlessness and wheeze. The prognosis in patients with clinically evident obstructive airways disease is worse than in 'simple' chronic bronchitis, and the two may well be different pathological entities. Patients with an FEV_1 of 50% or less of the predicted normal value have a particularly poor prognosis.

Complications

Complications of chronic bronchitis are responsible for the high mortality. The major complications are:

1 Respiratory failure.
2 Cor pulmonale.
3 Emphysema.
4 Polycythaemia.

Recurrent bronchial and pulmonary infections are very common and are usually considered to be inherent features of the disease itself, rather than major complications. Post-operative chest infections are a well-known problem in patients with this disease.

Clinical findings

Symptoms and signs

Clinical findings vary enormously, since there may be none in patients presenting only with cough and sputum, and at the other end of the disease spectrum there is the patient with features of all the complications (respiratory failure, cor pulmonale and emphysema). Hypoxaemic and oedematous bronchitic patients are often described as 'blue bloaters' in contradistinction to patients with emphysema who do not as readily develop respiratory failure and cor pulmonale — 'pink puffers'.

Before the onset of major complications most patients seek medical advice because of an acute exacerbation due to bronchial infection or symptoms of diffuse airways obstruction. The common auscultatory findings are inspiratory and expiratory rhonchi. Crepitations may be heard when excessive amounts of bronchial secretions are present.

By definition cough and sputum are features of all cases. Wheeze and breathlessness indicate chronic obstructive airways disease, or an acute exacerbation usually caused by bacterial infection. The presence of symptoms and signs of cor pulmonale (ankle oedema, raised jugular venous pressure and hepatomegaly), respiratory failure and emphysema indicate advanced disease of poor prognosis.

Finger clubbing and haemoptysis are not features of chronic bronchitis.

SLEEP AND SEVERE CHRONIC BRONCHITIS

In patients already hypoxaemic transient but severe worsening of hypoxaemia can occur during sleep. This phenomenon is particularly associated with the rapid eye movement (REM) phase of sleep and can cause an increase in established chronic pulmonary hypertension. The sleep-disordered breathing associated with exacerbation of hypoxaemia is mainly hypoventilation rather than sleep apnoea.

Radiological examination

Unless gross pulmonary infection, emphysema or cor pulmonale is present chest X-ray is usually normal.

Investigations

VENTILATORY FUNCTION TESTS

These may be normal in simple chronic bronchitis, but evidence of diffuse airways obstruction (FEV_1/FVC ratio of less than 75% and low PEF) is present in the majority of patients.

Exercise tests

The distance a patient can walk in a set time (e.g. 12 minutes) provides an accurate objective measurement of exercise performance. Response to treatment can be assessed by serial exercise tests.

LUNG VOLUMES AND TRANSFER FACTOR

Lung volumes commonly suggest the presence of emphysema (abnormally large residual volume and total lung capacity) and the transfer factor can be low in the presence of airways obstruction and is usually very low when emphysema complicates chronic bronchitis. Even if there are no abnormalities detectable by simple ventilatory function tests, assessment of small airways function usually shows abnormality.

BLOOD GAS ANALYSIS

Arterial blood gas analysis will show the presence of hypoxaemia, or hypoxaemia and hypercapnia in advanced cases.

ELECTROCARDIOGRAM

Evidence of right atrial and right ventricular hypertrophy is present in patients with cor pulmonale.

SPUTUM

Purulent sputum should be examined microbiologically for pathogenic organisms, particularly when there has been no response to 5–7 days' treatment with a wide-spectrum antibiotic (p. 38).

Differential diagnosis

The diagnosis of 'simple chronic bronchitis' is rarely difficult and in practice only bronchiectasis presents a problem. Tuberculosis and bronchial carcinoma have to be excluded, but in the majority of cases a straight X-ray is sufficient for this purpose. 'Chronic obstructive bronchitis' is sometimes difficult to differentiate from chronic asthma (*see* Table 2.1).

Table 2.1   Differences between chronic obstructive bronchitis and chronic asthma.

Chronic obstructive bronchitis	Chronic asthma
Rare or unknown in children	Common in children
Almost all smoke	Few smoke
Good night's sleep	Symptoms disturb sleep
Worse in the mornings	Worse at night
Cough on going to bed	Cough during the night
Cough and sputum in all	Cough and sputum in some
Exercise brings on breathlessness	Exercise brings on wheeze
Family history uncommon	Family history in young
Few respond to corticosteroids	Most respond to corticosteroids
Few have good bronchodilator reversibility	Most have good bronchodilator reversibility

Treatment

Bronchial hypersecretion

There is no satisfactory treatment other than removal of sources of bronchial irritation, usually cigarette smoking. The use of anticholinergic drugs to decrease sputum volume is contraindicated since they may also cause increased sputum viscosity which could result in worsening of symptoms.

Airways obstruction

Some patients with chronic obstructive bronchitis have a substantial reversible component, and in these patients the sympathomimetic bronchodilator drugs are of considerable value (p. 69). Ipratropium bromide, an anticholinergic drug with little or no effect on sputum viscosity, when given by inhalation (0·02–0·08 mg three or four times daily) is also a useful bronchodilator in patients with demonstrable reversible airways obstruction. Ipratropium bromide is also available in combination with a selective beta$_2$ agonist (fenoterol) in the same pressurized aerosol.

Unfortunately, airways obstruction in the majority of patients with chronic bronchitis is predominantly irreversible, and bronchodilator therapy is rarely dramatically effective. During exacerbations causing severe wheeze bronchodilator drugs should always be given. In addition, a trial of oral corticosteroids is probably warranted in all patients with chronic airflow limitation with severe symptoms. Long-term treatment with corticosteroids should not be used unless objective improvement has been demonstrated by formal assessment using exercise tests and/or ventilatory function tests (p. 25).

A small proportion of patients with distressing breathlessness benefit from high-dose bronchodilator therapy administered by nebulized aerosol (salbutamol or terbutaline 5–10 mg six hourly). Ipratropium bromide is also available as a nebulizer solution for such patients (0·1–0·5 mg four times daily).

Bronchial infection

The bacteria responsible for most infective exacerbations of chronic bronchitis are *Streptococcus pneumoniae* and *Haemophilus influenzae*. It is therefore important to use an antibiotic with an antibacterial spectrum of activity which includes both these organisms. *Branhamella catarrhalis* was until recently thought only to be an oropharyngeal commensal organism. However, this organism has now been shown to be pathogenic in some individuals and can be responsible for purulent exacerbations of chronic bronchitis. During influenza epidemics secondary infection with *Staphylococcus aureus* is common, and in such circumstances this possibility must be kept in mind when antibiotic therapy is planned. The decision to start antibiotic treatment must be made on the clinical features. All patients with an exacerbation associated with purulent sputum should be given antibiotic treatment, and it could be argued that all exacerbations should be treated with an antibiotic even though the sputum may be mucoid at first, since bacterial superinfection often rapidly follows an initial viral infection. Treatment must not be delayed until the results of bacteriological examination of sputum are available. Indeed most cases can be managed satisfactorily without bacteriology. Response to treatment should be assessed from the purulence of sputum, and the chosen antibiotic changed if there has been no improvement in the amount or degree of purulence of sputum after five days' treatment.

CHOICE OF ANTIBIOTIC

The vast majority of infective exacerbations can be effectively treated with one of the tetracycline drugs (the dose of the standard tetracyclines is 250–500 mg four times daily), ampicillin (250–500 mg three or four times daily), or one of its derivatives, erythromycin (250–500 mg four times daily) or co-trimoxazole (trimethoprim 80 mg and sulphamethoxazole 400 mg — two tablets twice daily). *B. catarrhalis* isolates often produce beta-lactamase, and infections with this organism are best treated with a tetracycline, erythromycin or co-trimoxazole, rather than with ampicillin or one of its derivatives.

Long-term antibiotic treatment is rarely justified, but many patients can be allowed to have a stock supply of a suitable antibiotic to be taken at an early stage of an exacerbation associated with purulent sputum.

MUCOLYTIC DRUGS, COUGH SUPPRESSANTS AND EXPECTORANT COUGH MIXTURES

These symptomatic remedies are rarely of therapeutic benefit. When sputum is particularly tenacious bromhexine (8–16 mg four times daily), carbocisteine (750 mg three times daily), or acetylcysteine (200 mg three times daily) should be tried in an attempt to decrease sputum viscosity. Potent cough suppressants (e.g. methadone) are potentially dangerous in patients with advanced disease and are contraindicated in the presence of ventilatory failure. The 'expectorant cough mixtures' are of little or no use even though they are liberally prescribed.

PHYSIOTHERAPY

Physiotherapy to aid expectoration is helpful in the treatment of exacerbations in patients with advanced disease. Simple 'breathing exercises' are of doubtful benefit. Assisted coughing performed by a trained physiotherapist is vital post-operatively and when elective surgical procedures are performed the physiotherapist should always be involved preoperatively at the earliest possible stage.

OXYGEN THERAPY

Whenever possible, continuous treatment with low concentrations of oxygen (24% or 28%) should be given during exacerbations to all patients with respiratory failure. This treatment is extremely important in hypoxaemic cor pulmonale in order to try to reduce pulmonary hypertension. The effects of oxygen therapy in acutely ill patients must be monitored by regular checks of arterial blood gases and pH (or hydrogen ion concentration).

Cor pulmonale (pulmonary heart disease)

The mainstay of treatment of right ventricular failure due to chronic lung disease is diuretic therapy. The selective beta$_2$ agonist bronchodilator drugs (e.g. salbutamol, terbutaline and fenoterol) may be of value because of actions other than bronchodilatation. These drugs may help in hypoxaemic cor pulmonale because they have a mild inotropic effect on cardiac muscle and might improve cardiac output. They can also decrease systemic and pulmonary vascular resistance. Digoxin (dose assessed for individual patients by clinical trial and serum levels) is indicated when there is evidence of co-existent primary cardiac disease causing dysrhythmias such as rapid atrial fibrillation.

A few patients with refractory cor pulmonale associated with secondary polycythaemia can benefit temporarily from venesection.

LONG-TERM DOMICILIARY OXYGEN THERAPY

Long-term low-concentration oxygen therapy (2 litres per minute by nasal prongs) has been shown to prolong life in hypoxaemic chronic bronchitic patients who have developed cor pulmonale. In the various studies of this form of treatment the best results were achieved when oxygen was given for more than 19 hours per 24 hours. This therapy is expensive, and if it is to be used the cheapest and most convenient way of administering long-term oxygen is by an oxygen concentrator. Selection of patients is extremely difficult because of the financial and ethical problems involved, but it has been suggested that patients should have an FEV_1 of less than 1·5 litres and be chronically hypoxaemic while awake and breathing air (arterial oxygen tension range 5·3–7·3 kPa). Excluded should be those who continue to smoke, as judged by a carboxyhaemoglobin level of more than 3%, and, of course, patients who cannot understand the controls of the oxygen concentrator. Treatment from oxygen cylinders and insulated liquid oxygen reservoirs should probably be avoided because of the high cost and inconvenience involved with these sources of oxygen.

Respiratory failure

See Respiratory failure (p. 77).

Prognosis

The prognosis in individual cases is difficult to predict. Patients without significant airways obstruction have a relatively good prognosis, and if bronchial irritation (cigarette smoking) can be reduced or removed the progression of disease may be arrested. When significant diffuse airways obstruction is established progression is usually relentless to death from respiratory failure and cor pulmonale. The single most important factor in prognosis is whether or not the patient can be persuaded to stop smoking before the onset of major complications.

SUMMARY — SPECIAL POINTS OF EMPHASIS

• There is no satisfactory definition of chronic bronchitis. The spectrum of disease extends from cough productive of sputum on most days during at least three months for more than two consecutive years to advanced chronic obstructive airways disease with associated cor pulmonale and respiratory failure.

• Finger clubbing and recurrent haemoptysis are not features of chronic bronchitis.

- Chronic bronchitis is very common and a major cause of death and prolonged disability.

- Cigarette smoking is by far the most important cause.

- Hypertrophy and hypersecretion of bronchial mucous glands are present in all patients, especially if the FEV_1 is 50% or less than predicted normal.

- Chronic diffuse airways obstruction indicates a poor prognosis.

- The major complications are type II respiratory failure and cor pulmonale.

- Recurrent bacterial bronchial infection and post-operative chest infections are common.

- Treatment is unsatisfactory.

- Progression of disease is usually relentless unless cigarette smoking is stopped before the onset of major complications.

- *H. influenzae* and *Strep. pneumoniae* must be assumed to be present in all patients with purulent sputum.

- Physiotherapy to assist expectoration is of vital importance in the treatment of all patients with advanced disease and in the prevention of post-operative chest complications.

- Reversible airways obstruction should be treated with a selective beta$_2$-adrenoreceptor agonist and ipratropium bromide by inhalation.

- The presently available mucolytic agents do not benefit many patients.

Further reading

Clark T.J.H. (Ed.) (1984) *Bronchodilator Therapy*. Auckland: ADIS Press Ltd.

Flenley D.C. & Warren P.M. (1980) Chronic bronchitis and emphysema. In *Recent Advances in Respiratory Medicine* — 2 (Ed. D.C. Flenley). Edinburgh: Churchill Livingstone.

Morgenroth K., Newhouse M.T. & Nolte D. (1982) *Atlas of Pulmonary Pathology*. London: Butterworth Scientific Ltd.

Chapter 3
Emphysema

General considerations

Chronic emphysema is characterized by increase in size of the air spaces distal to the terminal bronchioles and is accompanied by destruction of alveolar walls. It commonly coincides with chronic obstructive bronchitis but can occur independently. The causes of emphysema are the same as those of chronic bronchitis, particularly smoking. Cigarette smoke probably allows release of elastase enzymes from leucocytes in the peripheral parts of the lung and also inhibits antielastase properties of serum. These factors, together with the possible effects of smoke on surfactant and inhibition of alveolar macrophage and ciliary function, are likely to be the explanation, at least in part, of the genesis of emphysema. A minority of patients develop the disease because of inherited deficiency of the serum globulin alpha$_1$-antitrypsin, which allows excessive connective tissue proteolysis and the development of lower lobe emphysema at an early age, even in non-smokers.

Pathologically different types of emphysema can be recognized but the clinical presentation of each type is similar. Emphysema is also used to describe overinflation of lung tissue adjacent to atelectasis or after partial surgical resection of the lung (compensatory emphysema) and distal to partial bronchial obstruction (obstructive emphysema). Escape of air into the mediastinum and subcutaneous tissues is referred to as mediastinal emphysema and subcutaneous emphysema (surgical emphysema). Air trapping in asthma is sometimes called acute emphysema as opposed to the chronic irreversible state which is usually inferred from the term. Emphysema is more common in men.

Fundamental points of diagnosis

Clinical diagnosis of emphysema depends upon the demonstration of irreversible overinflation of the lungs. Radiographically the diagnosis can be confirmed by an abnormal peripheral vascular pattern and the presence of bullae. Computerized axial tomography (CT) can be used in the investigation of emphysema (*see below*).

Complications

1   Bullae, thin-walled air sacs lined by alveolar epithelium, occur in many patients with chronic emphysema. Giant bullae may compress adjacent lung and seriously impair already compromised pulmonary function.

2   Pneumothorax, caused by rupture of superficial thin-walled bullae, is a serious complication which is often difficult to treat.

3   Respiratory failure and cor pulmonale are generally late complications of 'pure' emphysema compared with chronic bronchitis, and patients may be very breathless but have normal blood gases — 'pink puffers'. Progression to death is usually rapid when respiratory failure supervenes.

4   Profound weight loss leading to emaciation is seen in some patients.

Clinical findings

Symptoms and signs

The predominant symptom is progressive breathlessness. A history of chronic bronchitis is found in most patients, but in 'pure' emphysema cough, sputum and wheeze may be absent.

Purse-lip breathing is characteristic of emphysema. There is marked air trapping in the hyperinflated lungs and purse-lip breathing is adopted in order to create a back pressure within the bronchi to aid expiration by delaying air trapping. The physical signs in the chest are wholly due to lung hyperinflation — barrel chest (Fig. 3.1), decreased expansion, decreased cardiac dullness and poor air entry. Rhonchi are audible in patients in whom emphysema is coincident with chronic bronchitis. Respiratory failure and cor pulmonale are found in preterminal cases.

Finger clubbing and haemoptysis are not features of emphysema.

Radiology

The radiographic abnormalities in emphysema are not easy to interpret, since simple acute air trapping simulates many of its features. However, absence of vascular markings in the peripheral third of the lung fields strongly supports a diagnosis of emphysema, and the presence of bullae is diagnostic. Bullae can also be found in patients with otherwise virtually normal lungs. Bullae in the lower zones favour a diagnosis of emphysema associated with alpha$_1$-antitrypsin deficiency.

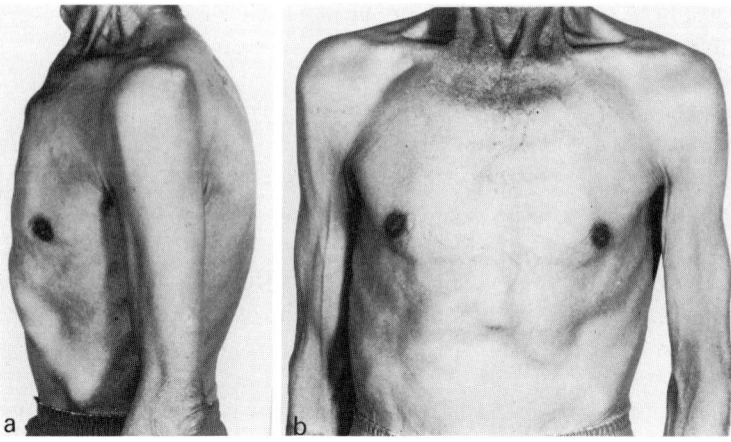

Fig. 3.1 Hyperinflated chest in emphysema (barrel chest).

CT scanning has been shown to be capable of suggesting the diagnosis of emphysema in patients without evidence of this disease on conventional chest X-rays. However, it is unlikely that CT scanning could ever become a routine procedure in the investigation of such patients.

Investigations

Ventilatory function tests always show an obstructive airways defect, but in some cases the FEV_1 and FVC may be remarkably good compared with the degree of breathlessness. In emphysema the relaxed VC is often greater than the FVC.

Transfer factor is usually much diminished.

Lung volumes confirm pulmonary hyperinflation.

Exercise tests.   The 12-minute walking test is of value in the assessment of functional disability and response to treatment.

Ventilation/perfusion radionuclide scans are abnormal in patients with extensive disease. Radionuclide scanning may be helpful in the investigation of localized emphysema when surgical treatment is being considered.

Arterial blood gas analysis is normal until the late stages of disease when hypoxaemia, and later hypoxaemia and hypercapnia develop.

Blood. Alpha$_1$-antitrypsin deficiency may be detected in a minority of cases.

Differential diagnosis

Progressive breathlessness may suggest a number of respiratory and cardiac disorders, but the diagnosis is rarely in doubt once the patient has been examined. Pneumothorax must always be kept in mind.

Treatment

There is no effective treatment. All patients should be encouraged to stop smoking. Bronchodilator therapy by conventional pressurized aerosol or nebulizer (p. 69) should be given to patients in whom a reversible component of airflow obstruction has been objectively demonstrated. A trial of oral corticosteroids should be given to all patients with distressing chronic breathlessness, but response to this treatment must be assessed by ventilatory function tests or exercise tests. Surgical removal or obliteration of giant bullae causing compression of lung tissue should be considered, but sophisticated measurements of regional ventilation and perfusion are necessary to select patients likely to benefit from surgical treatment.

Blood relatives of patients with alpha$_1$-antitrypsin deficiency should be screened and those found to have low alpha$_1$-antitrypsin levels should be encouraged not to smoke.

Prognosis

Rapid deterioration to death within a few years from respiratory failure, often without cor pulmonale, is the rule in young patients. In the elderly the disease appears to be relatively benign. Emphysema coincident with chronic bronchitis has a variable prognosis.

SUMMARY — SPECIAL POINTS OF EMPHASIS

• Emphysema means overinflation of air spaces distal to the terminal bronchioles.

• Chronic emphysema frequently accompanies chronic bronchitis but can occur on its own.

• Alpha$_1$-antitrypsin deficiency is a rare cause of emphysema.

• Respiratory failure and cor pulmonale are late complications of chronic emphysema.

• Purse-lip breathing is an almost constant finding in patients with severe air trapping due to emphysema.

• Finger clubbing and haemoptysis are not features of emphysema.

• Young patients with emphysema may have an extreme degree of weight loss.

• The radiological features of simple hyperinflation are not sufficient to make a diagnosis of chronic emphysema.

• There is no satisfactory treatment.

• Prognosis is poor in young patients.

Further reading

Morgenroth K., Newhouse M.T. & Nolte D. (1982) *Atlas of Pulmonary Pathology.* London: Butterworth Scientific Ltd.
Woolcock A.J. (1980) The pathogenesis of chronic obstructive lung disease with particular reference to the small airway hypothesis. In *Recent Advances in Respiratory Medicine — 2* (Ed. D.C. Flenley). Edinburgh: Churchill Livingstone.

Chapter 4
Bronchiectasis

General considerations

Bronchiectasis means permanent dilatation of the bronchi. The diagnosis can only be established by bronchography. It is usually acquired in early childhood as a complication of pneumonia — often pneumonia complicating whooping cough or measles, but foreign body inhalation and primary pulmonary tuberculosis are also causes (*see* Table 4.1). Bronchiectasis can ensue whenever bronchial obstruction is accompanied by infection in the collapsed portion of lung distal to the obstruction. Rarely it is congenital, as in Kartagener's syndrome, a triad of situs inversus, rhinosinus abnormalities and bronchiectasis. There has been renewed interest in these patients recently, since they have been found to have impaired mucociliary transport, thought to be due to ultrastructural defects of the cilia demonstrable by electron microscopy (Figs. 4.1 & 4.2). In adult male patients the spermatozoal tails have the same defects. Ciliary dysfunction leading to respiratory problems, including bronchiectasis, is not confined to patients with Kartagener's syndrome and should be suspected in all patients with unexplained progressive bronchopulmonary disease associated with recurrent or chronic infection. An association between chronic sinusitis, bronchitis, bronchiectasis and obstructive azoospermia has been described in patients who do not have situs inversus and have normal ciliary ultrastructures (Young's syndrome). As would be expected patients with mucociliary dysfunction almost always have additional problems with nasal sinus infection. Congenital hypogammaglobulinaemia and cystic fibrosis predispose to the development of chronic bronchial infection and bronchiectasis. Some of the causes of congenital bronchiectasis and

Table 4.1 Causes of acquired bronchiectasis.

Children	Adults
Pneumonia	Suppurative pneumonia
Whooping cough	Lung abscess
Measles	Pulmonary tuberculosis
Foreign body	Asthmatic pulmonary eosinophilia
Primary tuberculosis	Diseases causing extensive pulmonary fibrosis
	Bronchial adenoma

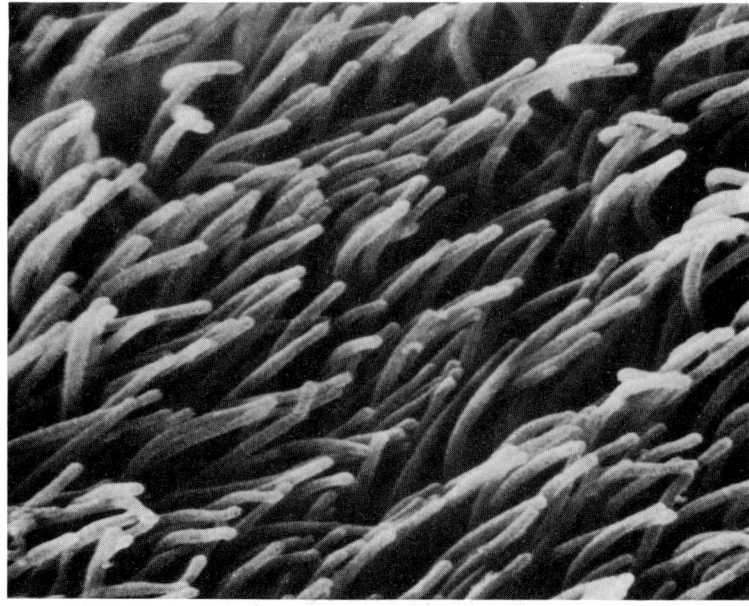

Fig. 4.1 Normal bronchial cilia. Bronchial biopsy examined by scanning electron microscopy.

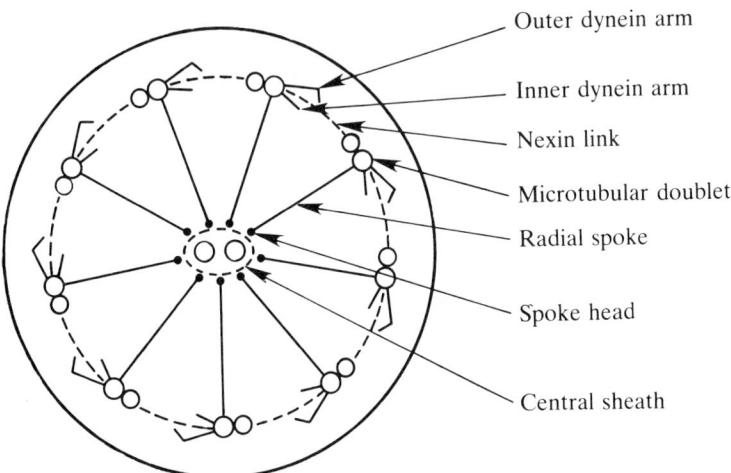

Outer dynein arm

Inner dynein arm

Nexin link

Microtubular doublet

Radial spoke

Spoke head

Central sheath

Fig. 4.2 Diagrammatic representation of the ultrastructure of a flagellum of a normal bronchial epithelial cell.

Table 4.2 Congenital bronchiectasis and congenital disorders predisposing to the development of bronchiectasis.

Congenital bronchiectasis
  'Ciliary dysfunction syndrome', 'ciliary dyskinesia syndrome'
    or 'immotile cilia syndrome' (including Kartagener's and Young's
    syndromes)
  Unilateral emphysema (McLeod's syndrome)
  Bronchomalacia (Williams–Campbell syndrome)
  Pulmonary sequestration
  Bronchial mucocele

Congenital defects predisposing to bronchiectasis
  Cystic fibrosis
  Hypogammaglobulinaemia
  Ciliary dysfunction

---

congential defects which predispose to the development of this disease are listed in Table 4.2.

In adults any disorder causing bronchopulmonary damage can produce bronchiectasis, notably post-primary pulmonary tuberculosis, suppurative pneumonia, sarcoidosis and asthmatic pulmonary eosinophilia. Sinusitis may occur with gross bronchiectasis but is usually an associated condition rather than a cause. The prevalence of this disease, which affects both sexes equally, is difficult to assess but was estimated as 1·3 per thousand in Great Britain in the 1950s. However, in the last two decades the improved treatment of childhood respiratory infections and the partial control of whooping cough and measles by vaccination programmes has led to a reduction in the number of patients with acquired disease.

Fundamental points of diagnosis

Frequently the symptoms and clinical findings (*see below*) allow a fairly confident diagnosis to be made in patients with gross disease, but the radiographic visualization of dilated bronchi by bronchography is the only certain way of confirming the diagnosis.

Complications

The complications of bronchiectasis arise from infection within the dilated bronchi.

INFECTION WITHIN A BRONCHIECTATIC DILATATION

Infection of bronchial secretions retained within the abnormal bronchi is the most common complication and causes cough productive of purulent sputum. Haemoptysis is common and may be severe. Bronchial arteries are larger than normal in bronchiectatic bronchi and ulceration of these vessels can lead to massive and sometimes fatal haemoptysis.

COMPLICATIONS DUE TO SPREAD OF INFECTION FROM BRONCHI TO LUNGS AND PLEURA

1 Pneumonia.
2 Pleurisy.
3 Empyema.

Empyema is rare, but recurrent pneumonia and pleurisy in the same site is a feature of untreated or poorly controlled disease.

COMPLICATIONS DUE TO DISTANT SPREAD OF INFECTION

Metastatic abscess formation, e.g. brain abscess (uncommon).

GENERAL EFFECTS OF CHRONIC INFECTION WITHIN THE BRONCHI

1 Finger clubbing is common in patients with extensive disease in whom bronchial infection cannot be adequately controlled.
2 Amyloid disease is now rare even in patients with extensive disease.
3 Stunting of growth. This is uncommon since gross disease is now rare and control of infection is easier to achieve except in patients with cystic fibrosis.

OTHER COMPLICATIONS

1 Pneumothorax.
2 Cor pulmonale.
3 Respiratory failure.
4 Fungal colonization of the bronchi and aspergilloma formation within bronchiectatic cavities.

Causes of death from bronchiectasis

1 Massive haemoptysis (rare).
2 Cor pulmonale.
3 Respiratory failure.
4 Secondary infection leading to pneumonia or septicaemia.
5 Invasive bronchopulmonary aspergillosis.

Clinical findings

Symptoms and signs

The characteristic symptoms are continuous cough and sputum. Sputum can be copious in extensive disease and is frequently purulent. Changes of posture, such as bending down or turning in bed, can elicit sputum production. A history of recurrent haemoptysis, pneumonia and pleurisy is relatively common. It is not rare for haemoptysis, even of a massive nature, to be the presenting symptom in patients with minimal disease. Breathlessness is a feature of very extensive bronchiectasis but wheeze is only present in patients with associated chronic bronchitis.

The most consistent physical finding is the presence of coarse crepitations constantly in the same site(s). Signs of collapse and fibrosis may be present. Finger clubbing is common in patients with persistently purulent sputum. In many patients there are no abnormal findings.

Radiology

The plain X-ray is frequently normal, but areas of pulmonary collapse and fibrosis are sometimes seen. Dilated bronchi, occasionally with fluid levels, only occur in gross disease. Otherwise bronchography has to be performed to confirm the diagnosis and is absolutely essential in the assessment of patients for surgical treatment.

Investigations

Ventilatory function tests may show a restrictive pattern in patients with pulmonary collapse and fibrosis. Airway obstruction is evidence of co-existent chronic bronchitis. Sophisticated pulmonary function studies may show evidence of arteriovenous shunting.

ASSESSMENT OF MUCOCILIARY FUNCTION

Patients suspected of having ciliary dysfunction should have tests of mucociliary function. The time taken for a small pellet of saccharin to travel from the anterior part of the nose to the pharynx, when it can be tasted, is a simple test. This should not exceed 20 minutes, but is greatly prolonged in patients with ciliary dysfunction. When facilities exist more specific tests can be performed. Ciliary beat frequency can be measured using small nasal biopsies taken under local anaesthesia, and the ciliary ultrastructure can be demonstrated by electron microscopy. Clearance of particles from the lungs, bronchi and trachea can be measured using radioactive techniques.

BACTERIAL EXAMINATION

Microbiological examination of sputum is necessary in the management of all patients with bronchiectasis. *H. influenzae* and *Strep. pneumoniae* are frequent pathogens, but colonization of the bronchi with other organisms is a common complication of prolonged antibiotic therapy. In patients with cystic fibrosis *Staph. aureus* and pseudomonas organisms are troublesome pathogens. Any patient, but especially those with cystic fibrosis, can develop *Aspergillus fumigatus* colonization of the bronchi, and aspergillomas may develop within bronchiectatic cavities. Regular mycological monitoring of the sputum (p. 118) is desirable and blood should be tested for precipitins to *A. fumigatus* every year or so in all patients in whom bronchial infection is difficult to control.

Differential diagnosis

Chronic bronchitis is the disease which is most often involved in the differential diagnosis and in many patients the two conditions co-exist. Occasionally pulmonary tuberculosis, recurrent pulmonary infarction and bronchial adenoma may simulate bronchiectasis.

Treatment

Postural drainage

The mainstay of treatment is drainage of secretions from the bronchiectatic spaces with the aid of gravity and chest wall percussion whenever possible. If postural drainage is performed regularly bronchial infection is rarely a problem, even in patients with extensive disease. Time taken in explaining the principles and details of postural drainage is never wasted. Ideally the abnormal bronchi should be drained twice daily for a minimum of 15 minutes and more frequently during exacerbations. The object of postural drainage is to position the bronchiectatic area of lung above the trachea so that secretions can drain by gravity, and chest wall percussion is performed to aid this process. Tuition by a physiotherapist should be given initially and whenever possible a relative should be taught how to perform chest wall percussion.

Antibiotic treatment

Long-term antibiotic treatment is potentially hazardous and is rarely necessary if postural drainage is regularly performed. Prolonged treatment with an antibiotic should not be continued in patients with persistently purulent sputum because of the almost inevitable development of drug resistance and the danger of superimposed fungal infection. Antibiotic therapy should be reserved for the treatment of exacerbations of bronchial infection causing constitutional symptoms, fever and increased sputum purulence and volume. The principles of treatment in bronchiectasis are similar to those in chronic bronchitis (p. 38). However, in bronchiectasis microbiological monitoring of sputum is more important because of the relatively common superinfection with pseudomonas and klebsiella species as well as *Staphylococci*. These organisms are usually found in patients who cannot be persuaded to perform postural drainage regularly, or who have cystic fibrosis.

Surgical treatment

Surgical resection of all dilated bronchi is the only method of relieving symptoms. The ideal patient for surgery has disease localized to one lobe or segment and with no evidence of chronic bronchitis or ciliary dysfunction. Bilateral resection in two stages was often performed in the past but is now rarely attempted because of the disappointing results. Unfortunately, surgery is not possible in the majority of patients with troublesome symptoms because of bilateral bronchiectasis or airways obstruction due to chronic bronchitis. It is, of course, imperative to assess all patients by bronchography and measurements of ventilatory function before contemplating surgery.

Surgical resection of localized unilateral disease in an otherwise fit patient is indicated when symptoms are not readily controlled by medical treatment, or if there has been massive haemoptysis or recurrent pneumonia.

CONTRAINDICATIONS TO SURGICAL TREATMENT

1 Bilateral bronchiectasis.
2 Evidence of co-existent chronic obstructive bronchitis — low FEV_1/FVC ratio and symptoms of wheeze and breathlessness.
3 Bronchiectasis complicating asthma (asthmatic pulmonary eosinophilia).
4 Evidence of ciliary dysfunction.

Prognosis

The prognosis of bronchiectasis has improved remarkably in the last few decades, but life expectancy is shortened in patients who cannot be persuaded to perform postural drainage regularly or cannot be treated surgically. Bronchiectasis caused by cystic fibrosis and asthmatic pulmonary eosinophilia has a worse prognosis than other types of disease.

SUMMARY — SPECIAL POINTS OF EMPHASIS

• Bronchiectasis means permanent dilatation of bronchi.

• Most symptomatic cases acquire the disease in early childhood.

• Bronchial obstruction and infection beyond the obstruction are responsible for the vast majority of cases.

• Abnormal ciliary function is responsible for progressive disease in a few patients.

• Symptoms and signs may suggest the diagnosis, but bronchography is necessary to confirm it.

• The complications of bronchiectasis are all due, directly or indirectly, to infection.

• Haemoptysis may be massive due to erosion of hypertrophied bronchial arteries.

• Finger clubbing is common in patients with persistently purulent sputum.

• Physical signs may be absent in some patients.

• Wheeze is not a symptom of bronchiectasis but indicates co-existent obstructive airways disease.

• The plain X-ray may be normal.

• Microbiological monitoring of sputum is important in bronchiectasis because of frequent colonization of the bronchi with organisms other than *H. influenzae* and *Strep. pneumoniae*, including fungi.

• Postural drainage is the most important treatment of bronchiectasis.

• Surgical treatment is possible only in patients with unilateral localized disease who have no evidence of chronic bronchitis or ciliary dysfunction.

Further reading

Afzelius B.A. & Mossberg B. (1980) Immotile cilia. *Thorax* **35**, 401–4.
Crompton G.K. (1982) Bronchiectasis. *Hospital Update* **8**, 914.
Goodchild M.T. & Dodge J.A. (1985) *Cystic Fibrosis: Manual of Diagnosis and Management*, 2nd Edition. Philadelphia: Baillière Tindall.
Hodson M.E., Norman A.P. & Batten J.C. (Eds.) (1983) *Cystic Fibrosis*. London: Baillière Tindall.

Chapter 5
Bronchial asthma

General considerations

Bronchial asthma is characterized by wide variations of intrapulmonary airways calibre over short periods of time either spontaneously or as a result of treatment. Diffuse narrowing of the bronchi causes an increase in resistance to air flow, especially during expiration, and produces symptoms of wheeze, breathlessness and chest tightness. It is very common and affects 1:50 of Caucasian races, but the majority of cases are mild and rarely require treatment. The onset can be at any age but the highest incidence is in childhood under the age of five. Although morbidity is high, mortality is low. However, the course of the disease is unpredictable, and no patient is immune from the severe and potentially fatal attack.

Atopic and non-atopic asthma

The asthmatic population can be broadly divided into those who produce excess IgE on exposure to allergens (atopic) and those in whom excessive IgE production cannot be demonstrated (non-atopic). Asthma in atopic individuals is often referred to as 'extrinsic asthma' as opposed to 'intrinsic asthma' in non-atopic patients. The majority of atopic patients develop asthma during childhood and early adult life, whereas asthma in non-atopic individuals develops mainly in adults (Fig. 5.1).

Atopic (extrinsic asthma) patients usually have a positive family history of disorders such as asthma, allergic rhinitis and infantile eczema.

Non-atopic (intrinsic asthma) patients do not have a family history of allergic disorders and because of the late onset of symptoms this type of asthma is often called 'late-onset asthma'.

Fundamental points of diagnosis

The diagnosis can be readily established from the history in the atopic child or young adult with a history of wheeze and breathlessness accompanied by other allergic manifestations, and by a family history of allergy. Sometimes, however, the correct diagnosis is not so readily apparent. Points of specific interest in the history include the following:

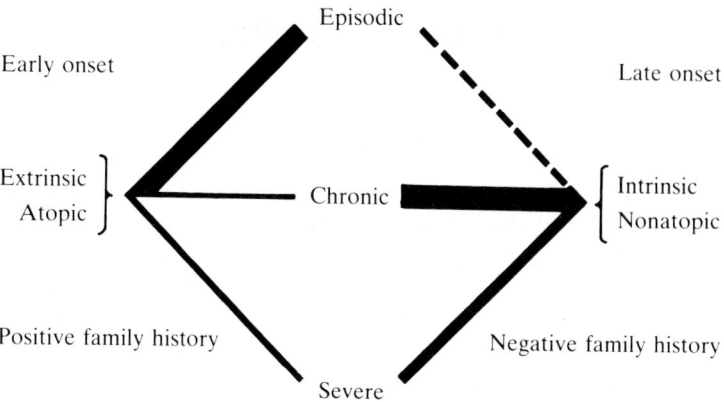

Fig. 5.1 Diagrammatic representation of the types of asthma and patterns of disease.

1 Asthma is often at its worst at night and many patients are woken by symptoms in the early hours of the morning (e.g. between 4 and 6 a.m.). Ventilatory function tests are at their lowest at this time ('morning dipping'). In contrast, patients with chronic obstructive bronchitis are rarely awakened by symptoms during the night.

2 Cough is a very common symptom of asthma. Nocturnal 'dry' cough is particularly troublesome in children, and in adults with chronic asthma cough is often productive of mucoid sputum.

3 Few asthmatics smoke during exacerbations, as cigarette smoke, and smoky atmospheres, may aggravate symptoms. In contrast, the patient with chronic bronchitis usually cannot stop smoking and may believe it helps expectoration.

4 In *episodic asthma,* episodes of asthma are interspaced with asymptomatic intervals; subjects are usually atopic.

5 In *chronic asthma* symptoms fluctuate in severity but are present continuously. Such patients may be atopic or non-atopic.

6 *Exercise-induced asthma* is common. Distressing wheeze and breathlessness can develop after completion of exercise and persist for about 30 minutes if not treated.

7 *Exposure to antigens* such as pollen, house dust, animal danders, drugs or foods may initiate symptoms within minutes. A history of exposure is not always volunteered and its detection may depend upon very careful questioning, particularly in the case of drugs.

8 *Other precipitating factors* include bacterial and viral infection,

inhalation of respiratory irritants (including smoke, dust, cold air and irritant fumes), treatment of other conditions (e.g. hypertension) with beta-adrenoceptor blocking drugs, and emotional upsets, though purely 'psychological asthma' is rare.

Status asthmaticus is an established term simply meaning severe asthma and serving no useful clinical purpose. Patients with any type of asthma can develop severe potentially fatal disease; the first attack can be life-threatening.

Complications

RIB CAGE DEFORMITY

Chronic asthma in children frequently causes thoracic wall deformity due to hyperinflation of the lungs and the effects of the muscular pull of the diaphragm on the lower ribs. Indrawing of the lower lateral ribs (Harrison's sulcus) and pigeon chest (pectus carinatum; Fig. 1.3a) always indicate severe chronic asthma, efficient treatment of which may result in reversal of the chest wall deformities. Hyperinflation of the lungs due to chronic air trapping in adults and older children can lead to a symmetrical increase in the anteroposterior diameter of the chest (barrel chest).

STUNTED GROWTH

Severe chronic asthma in children often causes retardation of growth.

PNEUMOTHORAX

Spontaneous pneumothorax is a rare but potentially fatal complication, and must always be excluded by X-raying patients with distressing symptoms.

MEDIASTINAL AND SUBCUTANEOUS EMPHYSEMA

Air can track from the lungs to the mediastinum and subcutaneous tissues of the neck, in the absence of pneumothorax, during severe acute asthma.

PULMONARY EOSINOPHILIA AND LOBAR COLLAPSE

A few asthmatic patients develop transient pulmonary opacities or areas of collapse associated with mucus plugging of the bronchi. The majority of these patients have an associated high peripheral blood eosinophil count and this syndrome is known as 'asthmatic pulmonary eosinophilia'. Such patients often have demonstrable hypersensitivity to *Aspergillus fumigatus.*

RESPIRATORY FAILURE

Hypoxaemia is present in all patients with severe disease but elevation of arterial carbon dioxide tension is evidence of disease which may prove fatal if not rapidly treated.

IRREVERSIBLE AIRWAYS OBSTRUCTION

Inadequately treated chronic asthma of many years' duration can lead to irreversible airways obstruction which may be indistinguishable from chronic bronchitis.

Clinical findings

Symptoms and signs

BETWEEN ATTACKS

There may be no abnormal findings but some patients will have chest deformity, nasal obstruction and eczema.

DURING AN ATTACK

General features

Increase in rate of breathing and prolonged expiration may be the only signs. During severe acute episodes fear and agitation are common and patients prefer to sit or lean forwards with fixed shoulder girdle muscles to aid the accessory muscles of respiration. Expiratory wheeze is audible without the stethoscope. Pallor, cyanosis and sweating may be striking features.

Respiratory features

Air flow obstruction is more marked during expiration and can quickly cause air trapping and overinflation of the lungs, leading to expansion of the chest with decreased cardiac dullness and depressed diaphragms.

During an episode high-pitched expiratory rhonchi with prolongation of expiration are consistent auscultatory findings over all areas of both lungs. As an attack abates, rhonchi become lower pitched and less pronounced. In very severe cases, there may be diminution of the intensity of the rhonchi due to extreme bronchoconstriction and physical exhaustion, resulting in very little air being shifted with each breath. Thus a 'silent chest' in an ill patient is of grave significance.

Patients with chronic asthma tend to have chronic cough and mucoid sputum. During an acute attack cough is a frequent symptom but sputum production is rare until the episode is on the wane or over. Secretions are retained because of bronchial narrowing and only released when bronchial calibre is increased. Occlusion of narrowed bronchi with viscid mucus is a constant post-mortem finding in patients dying from asthma. Mucous plugs and bronchial casts may be coughed up after acute episodes. Frequent production of bronchial casts is found in 'asthmatic pulmonary eosinophilia'. (p. 119)

CARDIOVASCULAR FEATURES

Increase in heart rate is caused by the mechanical effects of the abnormal intrathoracic pressure on venous return to the heart and by the humoral effects of hypoxaemia. Tachycardia is a valuable sign in the assessment of the severity of disease and should not be attributed to anxiety or the effects of drugs.

Profoundly hypoxaemic patients develop slowing of the heart rate and death may occur with cardiac asystole preceded by progressive bradycardia. A slow heart rate in an ill patient is usually a sign of potentially fatal disease. It is uncommon for patients to die suddenly from dysrhythmias such as ventricular fibrillation unless there is co-existent heart disease.

Pulsus paradoxus

Pulsus paradoxus reflects very high intrathoracic pressure swings and is a reliable indication of severe airways obstruction.

Blood pressure

Normal blood pressure is usually maintained during all but extremely severe episodes. Hypotension indicates potentially fatal disease.

Cyanosis and pallor

Clinically detectable central cyanosis is present only in severely ill patients and is often accompanied by pallor and sweating.

Cerebral effects of hypoxaemia

Hypoxaemia induces fear and restlessness, but patients are alert and orientated. Disorientated, confused patients should be assumed to have both hypoxaemia and carbon dioxide retention — carbon dioxide retention in asthma is a preterminal event.

Radiological examination

In the majority of patients the chest X-ray is normal or shows hyperinflation only. X-rays are essential in severe attacks to exclude pneumothorax and lobar collapse. They also provide the only reliable way of diagnosing mediastinal emphysema and asthmatic pulmonary eosinophilia.

Investigations

VENTILATORY FUNCTION TESTS

Measurements of FEV_1 and FVC will show an obstructive pattern (FEV_1/FVC ratio below 75%) and the PEF will be low in all patients with clinically significant airflow obstruction. Following administration of a bronchodilator drug the FEV_1 or PEF will usually improve by more than 25% in patients not in a severe attack or in remission (reversibility test). Ventilatory function tests are extremely valuable in the monitoring of response to treatment. Selected patients can be asked to record PEF regularly at home in order to document the pattern of disease and detect exacerbations at the earliest possible stage.

EXERCISE OR HYPERVENTILATION TESTS

The ventilatory function test response to exercise (5–7 minutes of vigorous exercise — treadmill, cycle ergometer, free running on the level or running up and down stairs), or isocapnic hyperventilation at rest, can help to establish a diagnosis of asthma, and by repeating such a test after treatment it can predict response to therapy (Fig. 5.2). A post-exercise

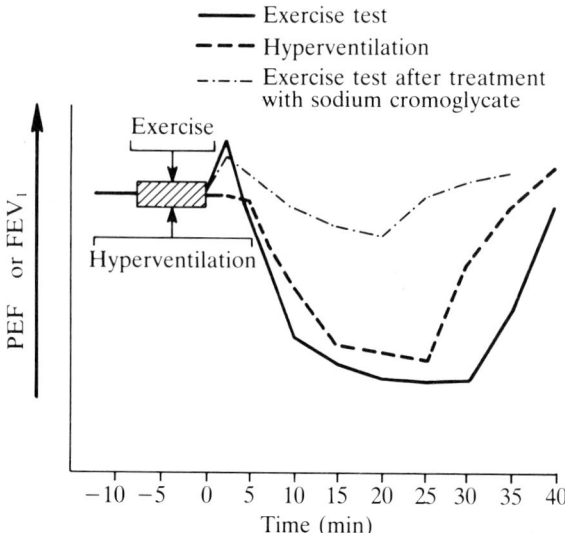

Fig. 5.2   Fall in FEV_1 following hyperventilation and exercise. Note small rise immediately following exercise, and almost complete blocking of post-exercise fall in FEV_1 by prior treatment with sodium cromoglycate.

or post-hyperventilation fall in FEV_1 or PEF or 20% or more is diagnostic of asthma.

SKIN TESTS

Positive skin tests (urticarial weal surrounded by erythema) 10–20 minutes after prick of intradermal administration of allergen indicates atopy. However, the significance of a positive skin test must be interpreted in the light of the history.

NASAL AND BRONCHIAL PROVOCATION TESTS

Nasal and bronchial provocation tests are much more accurate indices of hypersensitivity. Bronchial challenge tests using doses of inhaled histamine or methacholine can be used to demonstrate bronchial hyper-reactivity which is a characteristic feature of asthma, but these investigations are potentially dangerous and should only be performed in specialist units.

BLOOD TESTS

Arterial blood gas analysis

Estimation of arterial oxygen and carbon dioxide tension together with pH or hydrogen ion concentration is essential for efficient management of patients with severe asthma. A metabolic acidosis is not uncommonly found in ill children. Hypoxaemia reflects severe disease and the combination of hypoxaemia, hypercapnia and respiratory acidosis indicates an extremely severe and potentially fatal situation.

Blood eosinophilia

An increase in the absolute blood eosinophil count can help in the differentiation from chronic bronchitis.

Serum IgE and specific IgE

Elevation of total IgE supports a diagnosis of atopy, and measurement of fractions of IgE specific to one allergen can be useful in more definitive diagnosis but are rarely of more help than skin tests.

SPUTUM EXAMINATION

Sputum produced by patients with asthma often contains many eosinophils. Microscopical examination of stained sputum smears for mycelial fragments of *Aspergillus fumigatus* is essential in asthmatic pulmonary eosinophilia.

Differential diagnosis

Bronchitis with asthmatic features

There is no sharp division between asthma and wheezy bronchitis and the differentiation is often difficult. Most young patients thought to have wheezy bronchitis suffer from bronchial asthma. Separation of these diseases may be unnecessary since the treatment of both should be the same.

Stridor

Occasionally stridor due to an inhaled foreign body in children or a tracheal tumour in adults can simulate bronchial asthma, but stridor 'wheeze' is always more evident on inspiration.

'Cardiac asthma'

Episodes of left heart failure causing 'paroxysmal nocturnal dyspnoea' can simulate bronchial asthma since asthmatic symptoms tend to be more severe at night. Other features of cardiac disease usually make the distinction simple.

Pulmonary embolism

Very occasionally patients with pulmonary embolism develop broncho-constriction which is said to be unresponsive to bronchodilator therapy, but improved by treatment with heparin.

Treatment

There are two aspects to the management of asthma:

1   Day-to-day management to control and prevent symptoms.
2   Treatment of a severe acute attack.

Day-to-day management

The aims are to allow the patient to lead as normal a life as possible and to prevent severe attacks.

ELIMINATION OF NON-SPECIFIC AGGRAVATING FACTORS

General education is important and should include advice about smoking and avoiding smoky or dusty environments. Although anti-biotic treatment alone rarely influences bronchoconstriction, any bronchial infection probably requires prompt treatment with an appropriate antibiotic, and patients should be encouraged to look out for the first signs of sputum purulence. Likewise, attempts should be made to reduce emotional stresses, and in selected patients a psychotropic drug may be indicated.

AVOIDANCE OF EXPOSURE TO SPECIFIC ALLERGENS

In the minority of patients in whom the history and investigations reveal that a specific allergen is responsible, avoidance or reduction of exposure to the allergen concerned can bring about improvement. Unfortunately, such cases are few, and even elaborate attempts to avoid exposure to some allergens (e.g. house dust mites) are often unrewarding, nor is it possible to avoid exposure to allergens such as some fungi which are ubiquitous in the atmosphere. A change of occupation may be necessary in some patients, e.g. isocyanate-induced asthma.

HYPOSENSITIZATION

Hyposensitization (desensitization) by subcutaneous injection of increasing doses of extracts of the offending material has been used for well over half a century but there is little evidence that many patients benefit. Attempts at hyposensitization may be worthwhile in selected cases of asthma due to grass pollens, animal danders and perhaps, in children, house dust mite. 'Blunderbuss' hyposensitization with a number of allergen extracts should not be attempted.

ANTIHISTAMINE DRUGS

In general antihistamine drugs are of no value in the treatment of asthma. However, administration of one of these drugs at night may be useful in the highly atopic individual, but the therapeutic benefits are probably due mainly to the sedative effects. Antihistamine drugs with H_1-receptor blocking properties can produce bronchodilatation when given by inhalation.

SODIUM CROMOGLYCATE (SCG)

This drug modifies the antigen–antibody reaction. One of its actions is stabilization of the mast cell membrane and prevention or reduction of release of the humoral mediators of the asthma reaction. It must also have other properties not yet fully understood to explain all its effects, since many drugs which do not have the therapeutic properties of SCG stabilize the mast cell membrane *in vitro*. Its clinical effect is not confined to atopic patients since a few non-atopic asthmatics benefit from treatment. The drug is administered by inhalation either as a dry powder (20 mg four to eight times daily), from a pressurized aerosol inhaler (2–10 mg four to eight times daily) or as an aerosol from a nebulizer (20 mg four to six times daily). Its action is prophylactic and it is of no value in the treatment of an established episode. Its main use is in patients with chronic asthma or rapidly recurring episodic symptoms or in the control of exercise-induced asthma. Children tend to benefit more than adults but there is no way of selecting patients who will benefit from treatment with SCG other than by therapeutic trial for at least four weeks.

KETOTIFEN

It is claimed that this oral drug has similar therapeutic effects to those of inhaled sodium cromoglycate if given for prolonged periods to young asthmatics. Ketotifen has antihistaminic properties and causes drowsiness. The recommended dose is 1 mg twice daily to be increased to 2 mg twice daily, if necessary. The starting dose in patients known to be easily sedated should be 0·5-1 mg at night for the first few days.

CORTICOSTEROIDS

Corticosteroids are effective in the control of chronic asthma and are mandatory in the treatment of severe episodes. In chronic asthma, they are best given by inhalation in a therapeutically active form which is not absorbed in sufficient amounts to produce systemic side-effects:

Beclomethasone dipropionate (BDP) up to 1·5 mg per 24 hours
Budesonide (BUD) up to 2·0 mg per 24 hours
Betamethasone valerate (BV) up to 3·0 mg per 24 hours

Patient compliance can be improved, without decreasing therapeutic effect, by giving BDP or BUD in twice-daily doses, rather than the four-times-daily regimen first recommended for inhaled corticosteroid therapy. The only side-effects of inhaled corticosteroids when used in doses below those at which systemic effects (suppression of HPA function) are known to occur are oropharyngeal candidiasis (thrush), which is of clinical relevance in less than 10% of patients, and voice huskiness, which affects many more patients but is rarely more than a minor inconvenience. Huskiness or dysphonia is thought to be due to a reversible myopathy of the vocal cord muscles.

Corticosteroids for inhalation are available in the conventional pressurized aerosol (BDP, BUD and BV), in the pressurized aerosol with an extension mouthpiece attachment (BUD), or in a dry powder form (BDP) which is inhaled from a device similar to that employed for dry powder sodium cromoglycate. The spacer attachment to the pressurized aerosol and the dry powder inhaler are chosen for the many patients unable to use a conventional pressurized inhaler efficiently. Theoretically the extension tube device could lower the incidence of thrush, since it decreases the amount of drug deposited in the oropharynx. The large-volume spacers (Nebuhaler and Volumatic) substantially decrease oropharyngeal drug deposition.

Inhaled corticosteroids are of no value in the management of severe episodes of asthma when high-dose systemic therapy is essential (*see* Treatment of asthma, p. 72). A few patients with severe chronic asthma do not obtain adequate control of their symptoms with conventional doses of inhaled corticosteroids. It has been usual practice with these patients to add a small daily dose of oral prednisolone in order to achieve symptomatic control. However, an alternative is to increase the dose of inhaled corticosteroid as necessary and accept that systemic side-effects will result with long-term treatment. However, the effects of prolonged high-dose treatment with any of the presently available inhaled corticosteroid preparations are unknown. It is, therefore, probably safer to avoid such doses of inhaled corticosteroids and when necessary to add small doses of oral prednisolone.

Selection of patients for corticosteroid therapy

A decision to treat asthmatic patients with long-term corticosteroids should, whenever possible, be taken only after objective evidence of response to corticosteroid drugs has been demonstrated. Fig. 5.3 shows graphically an objective assessment which has proved to be very useful. This type of assessment can be undertaken in out-patients using a peak flow meter. Daily measurements of ventilatory function are made, preferably at the same times each day. Initially dummy prednisolone tablets (identical to 5 mg active tablets) can be given 4–8 times daily to

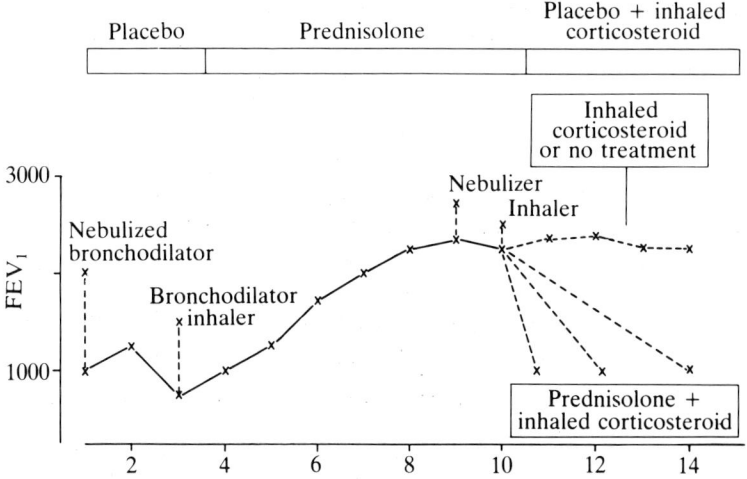

Fig. 5.3 Corticosteroid assessment.

eliminate any placebo effect. During this period reversibility tests to a bronchodilator such as salbutamol, terbutaline or rimiterol administered by conventional inhaler and/or nebulizer can be made. If spontaneous improvement is not observed after the first few days of placebo therapy active prednisolone tablets (20–40 mg daily) are then substituted and continued for at least a week. Response is monitored by increase in FEV_1 or PEF, and when this has reached a plateau active prednisolone treatment is replaced by placebo and at the same time an inhaled corticosteroid preparation is started.

Reversibility tests are repeated at this stage. Maintenance of the improved ventilatory function indicates that an inhaled corticosteroid drug alone should control symptoms, whereas relapse indicates that a combination of oral and an inhaled corticosteroid is required to achieve control. An improvement in ventilatory function of less than 25% in this type of assessment indicates that the air flow obstruction has not altered significantly and hence long-term treatment with oral corticosteroids is probably not indicated.

CORTICOTROPHIN (ACTH) AND TETRACOSACTRIN

There is no fundamental difference between the mode of action of corticosteroids and corticotrophin, though the latter requires to be given by intramuscular injection. Corticotrophin (initial dose usually 40 units daily and thereafter reduced in accordance with control of symptoms) has two potential advantages over oral prednisolone in the long-term treatment of chronic asthma:

1   In conventional doses it does not suppress the hypothalamo–pituitary–adrenal axis.
2   It does not cause as much growth retardation which is a serious disadvantage of long-term prednisolone treatment in children.

The need for treatment with corticotrophin and depot preparations of tetracosactrin (initial dose usually 0·5 mg twice weekly) has declined sharply since the introduction of inhaled corticosteroids. Corticotrophin is probably still indicated in the treatment of children in whom growth retardation has resulted from asthma or previous prednisolone treatment, but has little or no place in the management of adults with asthma.

DRUGS USED IN THE CONTROL OF REVERSIBLE AIRWAYS OBSTRUCTION (BRONCHODILATORS)

The most useful bronchodilator drugs are the sympathomimetic amines. Methylxanthine derivatives are of value in some patients. Anticholinergic bronchodilator drugs are of less value in the treatment of pure asthma than they are in chronic obstructive bronchitis. Although theoretically it should be possible to suppress asthmatic symptoms by regular treatment with bronchodilator drugs, in practice this is not possible except in mild cases.

SYMPATHOMIMETIC AMINES

In recent years selective beta$_2$-adrenergic receptor stimulants have been developed (salbutamol, terbutaline, fenoterol, reproterol, pirbuterol and rimiterol) and these drugs have replaced the less selective adrenergic agonists such as adrenaline, isoprenaline and orciprenaline because they have fewer cardiovascular effects. They are widely used in the treatment of bronchospasm and in the management of severe asthma. They are best administered by inhalation since this route of administration produces a quicker therapeutic response to a minute dose of drug compared with that necessary to achieve a similar degree of bronchodilatation when given by mouth. Side-effects such as muscle tremor and tachycardia are rare when these drugs are used by inhalation. They can be given regularly in an attempt to suppress symptoms or used as required when wheeze has developed. They are also of value if taken before exertion to prevent exercise-induced asthma.

Lack of response to an inhaled bronchodilator drug which has previously given rapid relief is a reliable indication that asthma has become severe and treatment with systemic corticosteroid therapy is necessary. Patients should be allowed to use bronchodilator inhalers as often as required providing they have been educated to seek medical advice if lack of response occurs. Many patients can be provided with a supply of prednisolone tablets and allowed to take this drug whenever lack of response to the bronchodilator inhaler develops, thus ensuring that corticosteroid therapy is given at an early stage of a severe attack.

High-dose domiciliary treatment with selective beta$_2$-adrenoreceptor agonists

In the last few years there has been an increase in the use of domiciliary high-dose bronchodilator therapy via nebulizer systems, usually using salbutamol or terbutaline in doses of 2·5–10 mg per nebulization. Large-volume spacer devices (Nebuhaler and Volumatic) have been designed for use with the conventional terbutaline and salbutamol pressurized aerosols. The Nebuhaler has been shown, dose for dose, to be at least as good as nebulizers in the treatment of chronic and severe acute asthma. Domiciliary high-dose treatment with any of the selective $beta_2$-adreno-receptor agonists must be used with extreme caution, since it is potentially dangerous in severe acute asthma, as undue reliance on nebulizers or spacer devices could cause the patient to delay seeking medical advice and thereby delay appropriate treatment (corticosteroids and oxygen). Whenever possible oxygen should be given during and after high-dose bronchodilator treatment.

METHYLXANTHINE BRONCHODILATORS

Aminophylline (5 mg/kg) by slow intravenous injection over 10–20 minutes is very useful in the treatment of the severely ill (*see also* p. 74). The dose should be halved for patients taking an oral sustained-release theophylline preparation in order to reduce the risk of serious side-effects. Sustained-release preparations have greatly improved the efficacy and decreased the side-effects of oral theophylline therapy, since they have made it much easier to achieve and maintain a thera-peutic blood level of between 10 and 20 mg/l. Side-effects such as nausea, vomiting and headache do occur with blood levels below 20 mg/l, but are much more common and potentially more serious (vomiting, hypotension, convulsions, etc.) when the serum concen-tration exceeds 20 mg/l. Ideally therefore theophylline therapy should always be monitored by repeated estimations of blood levels. Repeat checks are necessary because of the numerous factors which can alter the hepatic clearance of this drug (Table 5.1). A single dose of a theophylline slow-release preparation given in the evening can be successful in relieving nocturnal asthmatic symptoms which may not be controlled with $beta_2$-adrenoreceptor agonist therapy. The doses of a commonly prescribed sustained-release theophylline preparation are 800 mg for patients over 70 kg and 600 mg for those weighing less than 70 kg. During the first week of treatment it is recommended that all patients should have 400 mg once daily before the dose is increased.

Theophylline treatment is less flexible than inhaled $beta_2$-adreno-receptor agonist therapy, is responsible for more side-effects, and ideally should be controlled by blood levels. It should, therefore, rarely be the bronchodilator treatment of first choice, except perhaps in some

Table 5.1 Factors which can alter theophylline clearance.

Decreased clearance	Increased clearance
Drugs	*Drugs*
Cimetidine	Rifampicin
Beta-blockers	Phenobarbitone
Erythromycin	
Caffeine	Tobacco
High-carbohydrate diet	High-protein diet
Age	Youth
Obesity	Neuroticism
Liver disease or congestion	Alcohol

children who cannot use inhalers, but there is no reason why the two types of treatment should not be combined.

Enprofylline (3-propylxanthine) is a new bronchodilator drug with great potential since it is almost totally excreted by the kidneys and hence its clearance is not affected by the many factors which alter the liver metabolism of theophylline. Also, unlike theophylline, it has very little adenosine receptor antagonistic activity which is thought to be responsible for many of the side-effects of theophylline.

ANTICHOLINERGIC BRONCHODILATORS

Ipratropium bromide by inhalation is an effective bronchodilator but does not appear to have advantages over the selective $beta_2$-adrenoreceptor agonist in the management of asthma. It is available in a pressurized aerosol (0·02–0·08 mg three or four times daily) and as a nebulizer solution (up to 0·5 mg four times daily). The effects of long-term high-dose treatment on sputum viscoelastic properties and mucociliary clearance are not known. Ipratropium bromide has been used successfully in the treatment of severe acute asthma, but should not be used in preference to salbutamol or terbutaline, because it has a less rapid onset of action, and rarely bronchoconstriction may be induced by this drug. Ipratropium bromide should be used as a back-up treatment if a large dose of a nebulized $beta_2$ agonist has not been effective (e.g. salbutamol or terbutaline 5–10 mg), but can also be used in combination with such a drug.

The ipratropium bromide pressurized aerosol has little place in the management of patients with pure asthma, but is of value in the long-term treatment of patients with 'asthmatic bronchitis'.

COMBINATION THERAPY

It is often necessary to use bronchodilator drugs, sodium cromoglycate and/or corticosteroid preparations in combination to achieve good control of asthmatic symptoms.

Patient education

Patient education is vital in asthma, as it is in any other potentially fatal disease, e.g. diabetes mellitus. The minimum number of facts every patient should know about the disease and its management are:

(a)   Correct use of the inhaler(s).
(b)   The differences between inhalers and a full understanding of when each has to be used.
(c)   Diminished or lack of response to a bronchodilator inhaler means severe asthma which needs extra treatment.
(d)   The actions to take should a severe attack develop, e.g. seek medical advice, take prednisolone, etc.

Treatment of the severe attack of asthma

The essential prerequisites for the successful treatment of a severe episode of asthma are:

1   Early use of corticosteroids.
2   Early admission to hospital of severely ill patients whenever possible.

General practitioners should be encouraged to give hydrocortisone 200 mg i.v. whenever a patient with severe asthma has not rapidly responded to treatment with a selective $beta_2$-adrenoreceptor stimulant drug given by nebulizer or large spacer system (salbutamol 2·5–5 mg, terbutaline 5–10 mg), or intravenously (salbutamol 250 μg or terbutaline 250–500 μg) or intravenous aminophylline, 5 mg/kg or 2·5 mg/kg if on oral theophylline.

Whenever possible high-concentration oxygen therapy should be given during and after treatment with these drugs, since all are capable of temporarily increasing the degree of arterial hypoxaemia, especially when given intravenously. When admission to hospital is arranged the ambulance crew should be instructed to give oxygen during the journey to hospital.

Initial assessment and subsequent response to treatment must include:

Heart rate (preferably by cardiac monitor)

Measurement of degree of pulsus paradoxus

Arterial blood gas analysis

Chest X-ray (to exclude pneumothorax)

Ventilatory function tests — PEF

Serum potassium.

INITIAL TREATMENT

Oxygen

Continuous administration of high-concentration oxygen is necessary to improve arterial hypoxaemia. In practice a high-concentration Venti-mask is frequently used, since more closely fitting face masks are found to be uncomfortable by distressed patients.

Intravenous line

An intravenous access should be set up in all patients. This will allow correction of dehydration, but more importantly it will give a readily available intravenous route for drug administration.

Corticosteroids

Large doses are essential — i.v. hydrocortisone 200 mg loading dose and 1000 mg in the first 12 hours and/or prednisolone 20–40 mg loading dose and 100 mg in the first 12 hours.

Bronchodilator drugs

1 Selective beta$_2$-adrenoreceptor stimulants salbutamol or terbutaline are best administered by nebulized aerosol in oxygen. Intermittent positive-pressure breathing (IPPB) using a patient-triggered ventilator (e.g. Bennett or Bird) is often used but is not essential. A dose of 5 or 10 mg should be given initially. Alternatively these drugs may be given by intravenous injection (250 μg) or slow i.v. infusion (3–20 μg per minute). Salbutamol or terbutaline aerosol treatment can be repeated as necessary.

2   Aminophylline — by slow i.v. injection or the infusion of 0·5 mg per
kg per hour may be given as well as or instead of salbutamol or terbutaline. Theophylline blood levels should be used to monitor aminophylline
infusions (p. 70).

3   Ipratropium bromide (*see* p. 71). A combination of this drug and
salbutamol (or terbutaline) may be more effective than either drug
nebulized alone.

HYPOKALAEMIA

Serial measurements of serum potassium should be made during treatment since high-dose corticosteroid therapy and bronchodilator drugs
can cause rapid changes in serum potassium. Hypokalaemia, if present,
should be corrected rapidly.

The vast majority of patients respond quickly to treatment but
sometimes assisted ventilation using a powerful volume-cycled ventilator must be instituted via a cuffed endotracheal tube.

INDICATIONS FOR TRACHEAL INTUBATION AND ASSISTED VENTILATION

1   PaO_2 of below 6·5 kPa (50 mmHg) and falling.
2   $PaCO_2$ of above 6·5 kPa (50 mmHg) and rising.
3   Arterial pH of below 7·3 and falling.
4   Intolerable respiratory distress.
5   Hypotension — systolic blood pressure of less than 90 mmHg.
6   Cardiorespiratory arrest.
7   Severe exhaustion.

Prognosis

Mortality from asthma is low considering its very high prevalence. However, since all deaths are potentially avoidable and a high proportion of
fatalities are in patients under the age of 35, the present death rate is
unacceptable. It is not possible to predict the outcome in individual
cases. Although young patients usually outgrow their symptoms and the
disease tends to run a more chronic course in adults, a severe and potentially fatal episode can occur in any patient at any time. Treatment with
corticosteroids at the earliest possible stage of a severe episode and
prompt admission to hospital with facilities for respiratory intensive

care are the only secure means of preventing death from this unpredictable disease.

SUMMARY — SPECIAL POINTS OF EMPHASIS

• Evidence of atopy is readily demonstrable in many patients, but control of the disease by hyposensitization alone is rarely possible.

• All patients are potentially at risk of developing a severe attack.

• Exercise-induced asthma is common.

• Many factors can initiate an attack, but since the clinical end result is the same the treatment should be the same.

• Nocturnal exacerbations are common.

• Pigeon chest deformity in children reflects severe chronic asthma which demands vigorous treatment.

• Pneumothorax is a rare but potentially fatal complication of asthma.

• Hypoxaemia is a warning of severe disease, but carbon dioxide retention means impending death.

• Tachycardia indicates a severe attack and must never be assumed to be a manifestation of bronchodilator treatment.

• Progressive bradycardia is an ominous sign in an ill patient.

• Pulsus paradoxus reflects severe bronchoconstriction.

• Arterial blood gas monitoring of treatment is essential in all but mild cases.

• Control of chronic symptoms is most rationally achieved by inhalation of drugs such as bronchodilators, sodium cromoglycate and corticosteroids.

• Systemic corticosteroids in high doses must be given at the earliest possible stage of a severe episode.

• Tracheal intubation and mechanical ventilation are rarely necessary but must be performed in order to save life when the indications are clearly present.

• All deaths from asthma should be regarded as preventable.

• Patient education about the nature of the disease, the drugs used in its management and the recognition of the severe attack is absolutely essential.

Further reading

Clark T.J.H. (Ed.) (1983) *Steroids in Asthma*. Auckland: ADIS Press Ltd.
Clark T.J.H. (Ed.) (1984) *Bronchodilator Therapy*. Auckland: ADIS Press Ltd.
Clark T.J.H. & Godfrey S. (Ed.) (1983) *Asthma*, 2nd Edition. London: Chapman & Hall.
Lichtenstein L.M. & Austen K.F. (1977) *Asthma: Physiology, Immunopharmacology and Treatment*. New York: Academic Press.
Milner A.D. (1984) *Asthma in Childhood*. Edinburgh: Churchill Livingstone.
Stein M. (Ed.) (1975) *New Directions in Asthma*. American College of Chest Physicians.
Wilson J.D. (1983) *Asthma and Allergic Diseases*. Bristol: Health Science Press.

Chapter 6
Respiratory failure

General considerations

Respiratory failure can be defined as any condition which gives rise to an abnormally low arterial oxygen tension and/or an abnormally high arterial carbon dioxide tension. Usually cardiac lesions such as congenital abnormalities with right to left shunts are excluded. Respiratory failure can be conveniently divided into two main types:

Type I: Hypoxaemia without carbon dioxide retention.

Type II: Hypoxaemia with carbon dioxide retention (ventilatory failure).

Type I respiratory failure is found in diseases in which alveolar ventilation is normal or increased, whereas in type II alveolar ventilation is reduced. The term ventilatory failure is often used to describe type II failure. In general terms the conditions responsible for type I failure affect the interstitial parts of the lungs, e.g. pulmonary oedema, pulmonary infarction, pneumonia, fibrosing alveolitis and lymphatic carcinomatosis. The most frequent cause of type II failure (ventilatory failure) is chronic obstructive bronchitis. However, central depression of ventilation (e.g. drugs) and paralysis of respiratory muscles (e.g. polyneuritis) are other important causes. Acute ventilatory failure (asphyxia) can occur in laryngeal oedema and foreign body inhalation.

Although this classification is clinically convenient it is important to appreciate that death from any cause of respiratory failure is almost invariably preceded by carbon dioxide retention, that diseases usually associated with hypoxaemia without carbon dioxide retention may cause type II failure, and that airways obstruction does not always give rise to type II failure.

Fundamental points of diagnosis

The history and clinical features can be of great diagnostic help, but respiratory failure of mild degree is usually difficult or impossible to detect clinically, and arterial blood gas analysis must be performed whenever it is suspected.

Clinical findings

Although it may not be possible to differentiate clinically between the two types of respiratory failure it is usually possible to predict from the history the type of blood gas changes likely to be present in most cases.

Causes of acute type I respiratory failure

Bronchial asthma (unless very severe).
Cardiac disorders causing pulmonary oedema.
Pulmonary oedema of non-cardiac origin.
Pneumonia.
Pulmonary thromboembolic disease.
Allergic alveolitis.
Adult respiratory distress syndrome.

Causes of chronic type I respiratory failure

Fibrosing alveolitis.
Other causes of diffuse pulmonary fibrosis (p. 213).
Lymphatic carcinomatosis.
Thromboembolic pulmonary hypertension.
Chronic pulmonary oedema.

Causes of acute type II respiratory failure

Upper airways obstruction.
  Foreign body inhalation.
  Acute epiglottitis.
  Laryngeal oedema.
  Bilateral vocal cord paralysis.
Severe acute asthma.
Impaired consciousness and coma.
  Cerebrovascular disease, encephalitis.
  Drug overdosage (opiates, barbiturates).
Paralysis of respiratory muscles.
  Polyneuritis, myasthenia gravis, etc.
Pneumothorax.

Causes of chronic type II respiratory failure

Chronic bronchitis.
Emphysema.

Primary alveolar hypoventilation.

Most progressive respiratory diseases preterminally.

Symptoms and signs

TYPE I FAILURE

Respiratory symptoms

Hypoxaemia without retention of carbon dioxide is usually associated with distressing breathlessness. This is due to the underlying restrictive pulmonary disease but may be augmented by the hypoxaemia itself. In mild cases breathlessness is only present after exertion. Wheeze is not often a feature of this type of respiratory failure but asthma is an important exception. Symptoms of the underlying cause are often evident (e.g. cough and sputum in pneumonia, haemoptysis in pulmonary infarction etc.).

Central cyanosis

This is an unreliable but very important sign and indicates gross hypoxaemia with an arterial oxygen saturation of below 85–90%. The absence of cyanosis does not exclude significant hypoxaemia. Cyanosis is best detected by examination of the tongue in daylight.

Higher cerebral function

Hypoxaemic patients are alert, anxious and active. Fear and restlessness are common findings and confusion is found only in patients with profound hypoxaemia.

Extremities

The hands in type I failure may be cyanosed and cold since some causes (e.g. pulmonary oedema of cardiac origin and thromboembolic disease) may be associated with hypotension and poor peripheral circulation.

Pulse

The pulse may be of low volume and irregular — dysrhythmias may be present in cardiac disorders and thromboembolic disease.

In its classical form the alert, anxious, active and air-hungry patient with type I failure presents a completely different clinical picture compared with the patient with severe type II failure who is disorientated, drowsy, disinterested and has depressed ventilation.

TYPE II FAILURE

Most patients develop type II failure because of chronic obstructive bronchitis, but the other causes must not be overlooked (*see above*). The dramatic clinical features of carbon dioxide retention are usually only seen in patients in whom the development of hypercapnia has been rapid and is associated with a respiratory acidosis. In patients with chronic retention of carbon dioxide the respiratory acidosis has been compensated by renal retention of bicarbonate and the clinical picture cannot be readily differentiated from that found in patients with chronic type I failure without the aid of arterial blood gas analysis.

Respiratory symptoms

In uncompensated type II failure (respiratory acidosis) breathlessness, although usually present, is rarely as distressing as it is in type I failure, and is frequently associated with wheeze. Cough due to the underlying chronic obstructive bronchitis may be a conspicuous feature, but in severe cases it may be suppressed by the central effects of the abnormal blood gas tensions and acidosis. Inefficient cough with retention of sputum is a consistent feature of this type of respiratory failure in chronic obstructive bronchitis.

Central cyanosis

Cyanosis is usually present since physiological abnormalities severe enough to cause carbon dioxide retention almost invariably also result in quite gross arterial hypoxaemia and also because chronic hypoxaemia may itself cause erythrocythaemia.

Higher cerebral function

Higher cerebral function may be normal in patients with compensated respiratory acidosis, unless hypoxaemia is profound. In uncompensated respiratory acidosis cerebral function is often seriously impaired (carbon dioxide narcosis) where a striking feature is the apparent lack of distress in the presence of obviously severe disease associated with cyanosis. Drowsiness and disorientation are common and hypoventilation is often obvious.

Extremities

The hands, although cyanosed, are often warm because of the vasodilatation produced by retained carbon dioxide. In addition, many patients with uncompensated respiratory acidosis have the characteristic coarse irregular tremor (flapping tremor).

Pulse

The pulse is usually of high volume — bounding pulse — and regular.

The warm, blue and flapping hands together with a regular bounding pulse can often distinguish patients with type II failure from those with type I (cold, blue hands with low-volume pulse which may be irregular).

The fundi

Papilloedema may be present in patients with uncompensated respiratory acidosis.

Radiological examination

The chest X-ray may show one of the numerous causes of type I failure and hence aid diagnosis. In patients with type II failure associated with chronic obstructive airways disease and neuromuscular disorders the X-ray may be normal or show areas of consolidation or collapse, which often precipitate or complicate these conditions.

Investigations

The only investigation of real value in the diagnosis and assessment of type and degree of respiratory failure is arterial blood gas analysis together with measurement of pH or hydrogen ion concentration. Bicarbonate estimation is useful in the assessment of the degree of compensation of type II respiratory failure.

Serial arterial blood gas analyses are vital in the assessment of treatment.

Differential diagnosis

Respiratory failure is a complication of many bronchopulmonary, cardiac, chest wall and cerebral disorders and, therefore, the number of diseases involved in the differential diagnosis is enormous. However, there are also many conditions, not in themselves causes of respiratory failure, which must always be borne in mind. These include all cases of metabolic acidosis, salicylate intoxication, hysterical hyperventilation, methaemoglobinaemia, sulphaemoglobinaemia, etc. Respiratory failure must be considered in the elderly patient presenting with an acute confusional state.

Treatment

The principles of treatment in both types of respiratory failure are the same, but in practice this implies different management.

Principles of treatment

1 Treatment of the underlying cause.
2 Correction of hypoxaemia.
3 Treatment of the complications of hypoxaemia, e.g. polycythaemia, cor pulmonale, etc.

Type I failure

OXYGEN THERAPY

Oxygen can be administered in high concentrations since, in general, patients without carbon dioxide retention have normal central carbon dioxide responsiveness and hence there is no danger of precipitating respiratory acidosis. Indeed in most patients high concentrations of inspired oxygen are necessary to correct hypoxaemia. When there is no history of chronic obstructive airways disease and a normal or low carbon dioxide tension, oxygen masks designed to deliver low concentrations of oxygen should be avoided. When there is any doubt a reasonable compromise is the use of a 28 or 35% Ventimask until blood gas analysis clarifies the situation.

Type II failure

Table 6.1 summarizes the treatments of some of the causes of acute type II respiratory failure.

Table 6.1 Treatment of causes of acute type II respiratory failure.

Cause	Treatment
Upper airways obstruction	
Foreign body inhalation	Remove: Children — turn upside down and forcibly compress thorax. Adults — Heimlich manoeuvre. Laryngoscopy. Bronchoscopy.
Acute epiglottitis	Cannula through cricothyroid membrane. Endotracheal intubation. Ampicillin i.v.
Laryngeal oedema (infective)	Steam inhalation, oxygen, ampicillin. Tracheostomy.
Laryngeal oedema (anaphylactic)	Adrenaline s.c. Hydrocortisone i.v. Antihistamine i.v. Tracheostomy.
Bilateral cord paralysis	Endotracheal intubation — tracheostomy.
Severe acute asthma	Vigorous medical treatment (p. 72). If not rapidly effective endotracheal intubation and mechanical ventilation.
Impaired consciousness and coma	Maintain clear airway.
Barbiturate and opium alkaloid overdosage	Naloxone hydrochloride.
Reversible neurological disease	Endotracheal intubation and mechanical ventilation. Tracheostomy usually necessary.
Paralysis of respiratory muscles	Endotracheal intubation and mechanical ventilation. Tracheostomy at early stage.
Pneumothorax	Intercostal intubation and one-way drainage.

OXYGEN THERAPY

Oxygen therapy in patients with carbon dioxide retention is potentially dangerous, since once carbon dioxide responsiveness has been lost patients depend upon 'hypoxic drive' to stimulate ventilation. The administration of high concentrations of oxygen can remove the 'hypoxic drive' and result in worsening of the carbon dioxide retention and associated respiratory acidosis. Masks which deliver low concentrations of oxygen should, therefore, be used (e.g. 24% or 28% Ventimasks), or nasal prongs with an oxygen flow rate of 1–2 l/min and the effects of therapy must be monitored by repeated blood gas analysis. The principle of oxygen administration is to improve, but not to relieve completely, arterial hypoxaemia while other treatments combat the basic cause of the ventilatory failure — usually infection and retained bronchial secretions.

REMOVAL OF BRONCHIAL SECRETIONS

Natural coughing is the ideal method of getting rid of retained bronchial secretions. Physiotherapy is of vital importance to encourage and assist coughing, but to be effective it has to be performed frequently — even every one or two hours in severely ill patients. Unfortunately, many patients are incapable of co-operating because of drowsiness and impaired consciousness induced by acute respiratory acidosis. In this situation 'respiratory stimulant' drugs can be of value. These cerebral stimulants (e.g. nikethamide 25% solution 5–10 ml by slow i.v. injection) should be given intermittently to coincide with physiotherapy so that the patient is aroused sufficiently to be able to co-operate with the physiotherapist or trained nurse. Continuous infusion of so-called respiratory stimulants (e.g. doxapram hydrochloride 0·5–4·0 mg per minute) is probably as effective.

Therapeutic aspiration of bronchial secretions by bronchoscopy may be necessary in the comatose patient, or when a conscious patient cannot be encouraged to expectorate with the aid of a physiotherapist and a 'respiratory stimulant' drug. Bronchoscopic aspiration is mandatory whenever there is radiographic evidence of pulmonary collapse implying retained secretions.

Tracheal intubation, usually followed by tracheostomy, may be necessary in some patients to allow repeated bronchial aspiration by suction catheter and assisted ventilation. Assisted ventilation is necessary at the outset in totally unrousable patients with severe respiratory acidosis and in the majority of patients with respiratory failure caused by reversible neuromuscular diseases. Progressive deterioration of arterial blood gas tensions in spite of vigorous 'medical' treatment is the usual indication for tracheal intubation and assisted ventilation in patients with chronic obstructive bronchitis. However, the decision to ventilate patients with chronic lung disease is never an easy one. In general mechanical ventilation should be employed if the patient has recently been able to lead an active life, is young and the episode of ventilatory failure has been precipitated by an acute and reversible illness. This form of resuscitation should also be used in patients in whom no history is available, but if there have been previous episodes of respiratory acidosis and the patient has been severely incapacitated it may be merciful not to embark on such treatment.

MECHANICAL VENTILATION

Intermittent positive-pressure ventilation (IPPV) is used in selected patients with both types of respiratory failure. This is achieved through a cuffed endotracheal tube introduced through the mouth or nose under general anaesthesia. Positive end-expiratory pressure (PEEP) is used in some patients with type I respiratory failure (e.g. ARDS, pulmonary oedema, etc.) in an attempt to correct ventilation–perfusion imbalance. Volume-cycled ventilators are required for the treatment of patients with type II respiratory failure associated with severe airflow obstruction, e.g. asthma, and some patients with chronic obstructive bronchitis. If it is likely that IPPV will be required for more than a few days tracheostomy should be performed and the endotracheal tube replaced by a cuffed tracheostomy tube. Early tracheostomy is usually necessary in patients with respiratory muscle paralysis, e.g. infective polyneuropathy. Endotracheal intubation and tracheostomy allow tracheobronchial suction to be performed as often as necessary to clear secretions from the airways. This can be done efficiently under direct vision using a fibreoptic bronchoscope and is of particular value when there is radiographic evidence of lobar collapse. Retention of secretions frequently causes lobar collapse, particularly the left lower lobe, in patients being mechanically ventilated.

A ventilator volume of about 10 l/min is required by most adults to maintain a normal $PaCO_2$. The 'inspired' air is enriched with oxygen to achieve a satisfactory PaO_2. Ventilation with high concentrations of oxygen for prolonged periods should be avoided because this can cause ARDS.

As soon as the underlying cause of respiratory failure has been treated attempts to discontinue ventilation should be started. The patient is allowed to breathe humidified air spontaneously through the tracheostomy/endotracheal tube for longer periods each day until assisted ventilation is no longer required. In some patients with neurological disorders the tracheostomy tube has to be kept *in situ*, even though assisted ventilation is no longer required, to prevent aspiration of secretions when normal swallowing is not possible because of brain stem lesions.

High-frequency ventilation has recently been shown to be of use in some patients in whom conventional IPPV is inadequate. Various techniques have been used including high-frequency positive-pressure ventilation (HFPPV — 60–110/minute), high-frequency jet ventilation (HFJV — 110–400/minute) and high-frequency oscillation (HFO — 400–2400/minute). The place of high-frequency ventilation in clinical practice has not yet been fully established.

ANTIBIOTIC THERAPY

Most patients with chronic obstructive bronchitis develop acute respiratory acidosis because of respiratory infection, and treatment must include the use of an appropriate antibiotic (*see* Chronic bronchitis, p. 38).

Cor pulmonale

Many patients have cor pulmonale as a result of chronic obstructive bronchitis. This should be treated vigorously with a potent diuretic, e.g. frusemide (40–120 mg daily), and appropriate potassium replacement, together with controlled oxygen therapy. Cor pulmonale is often precipitated by ventilatory failure because of the increased pulmonary hypertension induced by hypoxia. Almitrine might prove to be of value in patients with stable hypoxaemic cor pulmonale since preliminary studies indicate that it can improve PaO_2 and $PaCO_2$.

Bronchoconstriction

The principles of treatment of bronchospasm in patients with ventilatory failure are similar to those in the treatment of the severe episode of asthma (*see* Asthma, p. 72), but selective beta$_2$-adrenoreceptor stimulants may also help patients with hypoxaemic cor pulmonale because of their effects on the heart and pulmonary and systemic circulations.

Prognosis

The prognosis of respiratory failure is obviously related to its cause. In many patients with type I failure complete recovery can be expected — e.g. pneumonia and thromboembolic disease — but the outlook for patients with cardiac disorders not amenable to surgical treatment is not so good, and the prognosis of patients with diffuse pulmonary fibrosis is grave once respiratory failure has developed. The prognosis of type II failure is also wholly dependent upon the cause. Respiratory failure in patients with chronic obstructive bronchitis carries a poor prognosis whereas many patients with type II failure due to neuromuscular disorders make a complete recovery.

SUMMARY — SPECIAL POINTS OF EMPHASIS

• Respiratory failure is present when there is an abnormality of arterial blood gas tensions (excluding low arterial carbon dioxide tension).

• There are two types of respiratory failure: (1) type I — hypoxaemia without CO_2 retention and (2) type II — hypoxaemia with CO_2 retention (ventilatory failure).

• Common causes of type I failure are pulmonary oedema, pulmonary infarction and pneumonia.

• The most common cause of type II failure is chronic obstructive bronchitis.

• Type II failure can be caused by central depression of ventilation and paralysis of respiratory muscles.

• Arterial blood gas analysis is an essential investigation in the diagnosis of respiratory failure.

• Patients with type I failure are often alert, anxious, active and air-hungry.

• Patients with type II failure are often disorientated, drowsy, disinterested and have depressed ventilation.

• The hands in type I failure are often blue and cold. The pulse is of low volume.

• The hands in type II failure are often blue and warm. The pulse is bounding and is usually regular.

• Clinical evidence of central cyanosis indicates severe hypoxaemia.

• Patients with type I failure need treatment with high concentrations of oxygen.

• Patients with type II failure can be made worse if treated with high concentrations of oxygen.

• Physiotherapy to aid expectoration is very important in the treatment of type II failure.

Further reading

Sykes M.K., McNicol M.W. & Campbell E.J.M. (1976) *Respiratory Failure*, 2nd Edition Oxford:Blackwell Scientific Publications.
Tinker J. & Rapin M. (1983) *Care of the Critically Ill Patient*. Berlin: Springer–Verlag.

Chapter 7
Pneumonia

General considerations

In clinical practice pneumonia is the term used to describe inflammation of the lungs caused by micro-organisms, usually excluding *Mycobacterium tuberculosis*. However, chemical, allergic and irradiation 'pneumonias' are often included in aetiological classifications of this common multifarious condition.

Pneumonia can be classified anatomically as lobar, segmental or lobular (bronchopneumonia), or aetiologically according to the causal organism (primary pneumonia). On occasions commensal organisms, or organisms normally of low virulence, cause pulmonary infection in susceptible patients (secondary pneumonia). Pneumonia can, therefore, be split into two main types:

1 Primary pneumonia or specific pneumonia.
2 Secondary pneumonia or aspiration pneumonia.

Primary pneumonia can be conveniently divided into two main subgroups:

(a) Bacterial pneumonia.
(b) Pneumonia caused by other organisms, e.g. virus, mycoplasma, chlamydia, coxiella, legionella, fungus and protozoa.

Secondary pneumonia and aspiration pneumonia are terms used to describe pulmonary infections which develop because of predisposing factors such as depression of the cough mechanism allowing aspiration of infected material from the upper respiratory tract, e.g. hypostatic and post-operative pneumonia. These pneumonias are often found to be caused by organisms normally of low virulence.

Most patients are effectively treated in their own homes. The common medical reasons for hospital treatment are:

(a) Very young or elderly patients.
(b) Severe initial illness.
(c) Co-existent chronic bronchitis, bronchiectasis, neurological disorder, etc.
(d) Suspected complications.
(e) Lack of response to treatment.
(f) Pneumonia in immunocompromised patients.

Fundamental points of diagnosis

Bacterial pneumonias often produce a characteristic clinical picture of sudden illness associated with pyrexia and cough productive of purulent sputum. The diagnosis can often be confirmed by the presence of grossly abnormal physical signs and X-ray changes. However, non-bacterial pulmonary infections often produce clinical syndromes, unlike the bacterial pneumonias, and the 'atypical' features of these infections often leads to the clinical suspicion that the offending organism is not a bacterium. The term 'primary atypical pneumonia' was used to describe the atypical clinical features of mycoplasmal pneumonia compared with 'typical' pneumococcal pneumonia.

Complications

Complications are most often seen in bacterial pneumonias. Bacterial pneumonia itself is often a complication of pulmonary infections caused by other organisms, especially viruses. The most common complications of pneumonia are:

1 Pleural effusion.
2 Empyema.
3 Lung abscess.
4 Pulmonary collapse (atelectasis).
5 Respiratory failure.
6 Cor pulmonale.
7 Pneumothorax.
8 Septicaemia.
9 Herpes labialis.
10 Thromboembolic disease.

Pleural effusion often complicates bacterial pneumonia and can be the cause of persisting pyrexia in spite of adequate antibiotic treatment or the recurrence of pyrexia during treatment. Empyema is rare and is now only seen in patients in whom appropriate antibiotic therapy has been delayed or when the development of a pleural effusion has not been recognized. Lung abscess is a frequent complication of bacterial infections due to organisms other than *Strep. pneumoniae*. Pulmonary collapse is rarely seen except in desperately ill patients who cannot cough efficiently and retained secretions cause bronchial obstruction. Hypoxaemia (type I respiratory failure) is found in all but very mild cases of pneumonia and even trivial pulmonary infection can precipitate type II respiratory failure in patients with chronic obstructive bronchitis. Clinical evidence of right ventricular failure may appear for the first time during an episode of pneumonia in a patient with chronic lung disease. Established cor pulmonale is always made worse by the insult of pulmonary infection and its associated hypoxaemia.

Septicaemia is a serious complication of staphylococcal infections and pneumonias due to Gram-negative organisms unless effective antibiotic therapy is started early. Bacteraemia can be detected in the initial stages of the majority of cases of pneumococcal pneumonia.

Herpes labialis (herpes simplex virus) complicates pneumococcal pneumonia so frequently that its presence in a patient with respiratory symptoms provides a diagnostically valuable physical sign.

Peripheral venous thrombosis and pulmonary thromboembolism undoubtedly complicate pneumonia. However, it is likely that in the past the frequency of these complications has been exaggerated since pulmonary infarction often simulates pneumonia (*see* Pulmonary thromboembolism).

Rare complications of pneumonia of various aetiologies are meningism (especially in children), jaundice, haemolytic anaemia, pericarditis, myocarditis, cerebellar ataxia, peripheral neuropathy, glomerulonephritis and generalized lymphadenopathy.

Clinical findings

The clinical features of pneumonia vary considerably according to its cause and severity. Since pneumococcal pneumonia is the most common its clinical features will be considered first and then compared with other types of pneumonia.

Pneumococcal pneumonia

SYMPTOMS

The onset is usually sudden but is often preceded by symptoms of an upper respiratory tract infection (common cold). The initial symptoms are due to rapid development of a high pyrexia (up to 40°C) which may induce a rigor. Profound prostration accompanied by non-specific symptoms of pyrexia may be the only features initially, and pulmonary disease may not be suspected at this stage. Frequently, however, pleuritic pain develops early, and the association of pyrexia and pleuritic pain, especially when preceded by an upper respiratory tract infection, allows the diagnosis of pneumonia to be made with some confidence from the history alone. Cough may be absent or unproductive during the first 24 hours or so. After a few days, sputum, which often has a characteristic rusty colour, becomes a conspicuous feature. The development of herpes labialis, which may extend from the lips to the nose and nostrils, is common enough to be used as a diagnostic sign.

The severity of the disease is extremely variable. Some patients with extensive disease are desperately ill and may be profoundly hypoxaemic, disorientated and hypotensive, whereas others may be so mildly upset that the condition may go unrecognized and simply be thought to be a bad cold. Type 3 pneumococcus tends to cause more serious disease than other serotypes.

CLINICAL FINDINGS

Pyrexia may be associated with rigors and herpes labialis. Most patients appear flushed and miserable. Cyanosis and hypotension are found in those with overwhelming infection or in patients with co-existent chronic cardiorespiratory disease. The respiratory rate is rapid and breathing shallow, particularly in patients with pleuritic pain.

The physical signs in the chest vary according to the stage and extent of the disease:

Early, before consolidation has developed

There may be slight reduction in chest expansion over the affected area of lung but this is often difficult to elicit. Percussion note is impaired. Auscultation may reveal slight diminution of normal breath sounds together with inspiratory fine crepitations.

When lobar consolidation is established

Consolidation usually develops about 48 hours after the onset of symptoms and when fully established produces the characteristic clinical abnormalities of:

1 Decreased chest expansion.
2 Dull percussion note.
3 High-pitched bronchial breath sounds.
4 Increased vocal resonance (whispering pectoriloquy).

As consolidation is resolving

Bronchial breathing may still be audible but it is of lower pitch and rapidly becomes replaced by normal breath sounds accompanied by numerous coarse crepitations. The crepitations disappear as the consolidation resolves.

A pleural friction rub may be audible even in the absence of pleuritic pain. In patients with severe pleuritic pain pleural friction may not be heard because of shallow breathing induced by pain.

The development of complications such as pleural effusion or pulmonary collapse considerably alters the clinical findings.

Other bacterial pneumonias

Pneumonia may be caused by many bacteria other than *Strep. pneumoniae*, but the most important organisms are *Staphylococcus aureus, Klebsiella pneumoniae, Pseudomonas pyocyanea* or *aeruginosa* and *Haemophilus influenzae*. Pneumonia caused by these organisms differs in many respects from classical pneumococcal pneumonia. Whereas a pneumococcal infection is common in previously healthy patients, *Staph. aureus* and the Gram-negative bacteria usually only cause pulmonary infection in patients with a predisposing factor such as diabetes, alcoholism, tracheostomy, chronic bronchitis, bronchiectasis, cystic fibrosis and immune-deficiency states due to disease or drugs. Staphylococcal pneumonia is also a serious complication of influenza. These organisms may produce lobar consolidation and hence similar physical signs to those of pneumococcal pneumonia. However, pulmonary suppuration and destruction leading to abscess formation are much more common, and this is reflected clinically by the production of copious amounts of purulent sputum which may be foul-smelling and sometimes dark-brown in colour. Haemoptysis is very much more common when pulmonary suppuration and abscess formation occur.

The physical signs in the chest in lobular pneumonia (bronchopneu-monia) are frequently difficult to detect. The most consistent finding is the presence of inspiratory crepitations.

Legionnaires' disease

This name was adopted following an outbreak of pneumonia with a high death rate among American legionnaires attending a convention in

Philadelphia in 1976. It has since been recognized in many countries and it is now clear that milder forms of the disease occur and that sporadic cases are quite common. Presently there are five recognized legionella species and six serogroups of *L. pneumophila*. The organism is a weakly staining Gram-negative rod, which is sometimes flagellated. It has been isolated from shower heads and air-conditioning systems. Inhalation of water droplets, possibly containing living organisms ingested by amoebae, has been postulated as the route of infection. Direct infection from human to human does not appear to occur, although pathologists may be at risk while performing autopsies.

Clinical features include a 'viral-type' illness, often associated with headache and marked confusion. Central nervous system dysfunction and peripheral neuropathy have been reported as manifestations of the disease, as well as abdominal distension and diarrhoea. Hyponatraemia, hypoalbuminaemia, abnormal liver function tests, lymphopenia and moderate leucocytosis are common laboratory findings. The chest X-ray can show lobar consolidation or bronchopneumonic shadowing, both of which can be bilateral and associated with small pleural effusions.

The diagnosis of legionnaires' disease is frequently suspected on clinical grounds because of the profound constitutional upset and marked confusion. Confirmation of the diagnosis can be achieved by Dieterle's staining, immunofluorescence or electron microscopy. Response to treatment is rarely dramatic. Most patients slowly recover but some are left with considerable pulmonary destruction and fibrosis.

Pneumonia due to viruses, chlamydiae, coxiellae and *Mycoplasma pneumoniae*

The clinical features of viral, chlamydial (psittacosis), coxiella (Q fever) and mycoplasmal pneumonia are similar and can be described together. All can be complicated by bacterial superinfection which can rapidly alter the clinical picture. In general the onset of symptoms is less dramatic than in pneumococcal pneumonia, and constitutional symptoms of lethargy, headache, arthralgia and fever may precede respiratory symptoms by many days. The presence of the pneumonia may only be detected by radiological examination of the chest. When they occur respiratory symptoms are seldom dramatic, except in rare fulminating cases of influenza, psittacosis and mycoplasmal pneumonia. Cough is common but is usually unproductive or sputum is scanty and mucoid. Blood-stained sputum is seen only in very severe infection. Pleuritic pain is uncommon. Wheeze may be a feature of viral pneumonia in young children (e.g. respiratory syncytial virus). Breathlessness indicates massive pulmonary involvement and is uncommon except in young children, when airways obstruction due to widespread 'bronchiolitis' complicates the picture. Varicella (chickenpox) in adults can be accompanied by severe lobular pneumonia which may leave permanent miliary calcification. In mycoplasmal pneumonia the symptoms may more closely resemble bacterial pneumonia but systemic symptoms such as arthralgia, headache and earache are usually more prominent than in bacterial infections.

These pneumonias often occur in outbreaks in institutions such as nurseries, schools and military camps. In the case of psittacosis there may be a history of contact with birds, and in Q fever there is often a history of contact with animals, e.g. abattoir workers.

The physical signs vary enormously. It is common to find no abnormalities even though the X-ray may show considerable changes. Lobar consolidation is much less frequent than in bacterial pneumonia and usually the clinical abnormalities are those of lobular pneumonia (bronchopneumonia).

Fungal pneumonias

Fungal pneumonia is rare in Britain but it is becoming more common because of immunosuppressive therapy and the excessive use of widespectrum antibiotics. In certain parts of the world, however, infections with *Histoplasma capsulatum* and *Coccidioides immitis* are frequent.

HISTOPLASMOSIS

Primary pulmonary histoplasmosis is often asymptomatic. Occasionally it is accompanied by mild febrile symptoms, and very occasionally it causes chest pain, cough and haemoptysis. Acute progressive histoplasmosis produces a commonly fatal disease which is similar clinically and radiographically to miliary tuberculosis. The chronic progressive form of this disease simulates chronic pulmonary tuberculosis.

COCCIDIOIDOMYCOSIS

Coccidioidomycosis also has two forms — primary and progressive. Primary coccidioidomycosis behaves very much like primary tuberculosis or histoplasmosis and often does not produce recognizable symptoms. The progressive form of the disease is associated with marked systemic upset and respiratory symptoms and signs of lobular pneumonia. In more chronic cases granulomatous lesions develop within the lungs and can be responsible for symptoms resembling chronic tuberculosis.

Aspergillus fumigatus pneumonia is rare but serious (*see* Invasive pulmonary aspergillosis). Pulmonary candidiasis is also rare, but can occur in immunosuppressed patients and also as a complication of prolonged wide-spectrum antibiotic treatment. It has no specific features and diagnosis is often difficult. Yeasts are commonly cultured from sputum of patients with bacterial pneumonia being treated with antibiotics and hence a positive culture for *Candida albicans* on its own is never diagnostic.

Protozoal pneumonias

Toxoplasmosis (Toxoplasma gondii) is a universal disease but uncommon in developed countries. Infection is usually acquired from domestic animals, but occasionally is congenital. In some cases of acquired toxoplasmosis respiratory symptoms, which may be similar to those of influenza, can occur and there may be clinical and X-ray signs of patchy areas of consolidation. *Pneumocystis carinii,* an organism which is probably a protozoon, but regarded by some to be a fungus, occurs in a wide variety of animals and has long been known to be the cause of pneumonia in the newborn. Pulmonary infection in adults is becoming more common as a result of immunosuppressive therapy. Recently, *Pneumocystis carinii* pneumonia has had much publicity because of its association with other infections and Kaposi's sarcoma in the acquired immune deficiency syndrome (AIDS) which is an increasing problem in homosexual men, drug addicts and those patients with blood disorders requiring repeated blood transfusions. The diagnosis is difficult without histological proof but infection with *Pneumocystis carinii* must be considered in any immunosuppressed patient, homosexual or drug addict with pneumonia for which no other cause has been found and antibiotic treatment has been ineffective.

Viral and non-bacterial pneumonias are summarized in Table 7.1.

Radiological examination

The diagnosis of pneumonia should be confirmed radiologically and response to treatment assessed by serial X-rays. Pneumonia can produce

Table 7.1 Viral and non-bacterial pneumonias.

Organism	Treatment
Viruses	
Influenza	—
Varicella	—
Cytomegalovirus	—
Adenovirus (3,4,7,14,21)	—
Measles	—
Respiratory syncytial	—
Chlamydiae	
Chlamydia psittaci (psittacosis)	Tetracycline/penicillin
Chlamydia trachomatis	Erythromycin
Coxiellae	
Coxiella burnetii (Q fever)	Tetracycline/erythromycin/ co-trimoxazole/rifampicin
Protozoa	
Pneumocystis carinii	Co-trimoxazole/pentamidine
Toxoplasma gondii	Sulphonamide + pyrimethamine
Fungi	
Aspergillus fumigatus	Amphotericin + flucytosine
Candida albicans	Amphotericin + flucytosine
Histoplasma capsulatum	Amphotericin, ? ketaconazole
Coccidioides immitis	Amphotericin, ? ketaconazole
Others	
Legionella pneumophila	Erythromycin + rifampicin
Mycoplasma pneumoniae	Tetracycline/erythromycin

many different radiological abnormalities and it is not possible to make an aetiological diagnosis from the X-ray alone. The common radiological changes seen in pneumonia are:

1 Consolidation.
2 Consolidation with abscess formation.
3 Multiple abscesses.
4 Lobular shadowing.
5 Miliary shadowing.
6 Pulmonary collapse.
7 Pleural effusion.

Consolidation seen on the X-ray as confluent shadowing may be confined to a segment, lobe or lung. In consolidation without collapse there is no evidence of shrinkage of lung tissue (Fig. 7.1a). Abscess formation usually indicates the presence of infection with bacteria other than *Strep. pneumoniae* (Fig. 7.1b). Multiple abscesses occur in staphylococcal pneumonia especially in children. Lobular shadowing may be confined to a lobe or segment, or be extensive and bilateral. Lobular shadowing is somewhat more common in the lower lobes than in the upper lobes. Miliary shadowing can be present in all types of pneumonia and is a relatively common feature of some of the fungal infections. Pulmonary collapse (Fig. 7.1c) may be a complication of pneumonia when sputum obstructs a major bronchus, but usually evidence of collapse, especially in a patient who is not severely ill and can cough efficiently, should raise the suspicion that the pneumonia is a complication of bronchial carcinoma. Pleural effusion (p. 164) commonly complicates bacterial pneumonia, and small effusions, not evident clinically, are often detected radiologically.

In all patients it is important to repeat the chest X-ray at intervals to ensure that satisfactory resolution has occurred.

Investigations

SPUTUM

Bacteriological examination of sputum is important in all ill patients with pneumonia, providing the sputum is purulent. Culture of mucoid sputum may give clinically misleading results. Also, no pathogens may be cultured from grossly purulent sputum. This is particularly common in cases of pneumococcal pneumonia if the sputum specimen is taken after antibiotic therapy has been started. In the severely ill, Gram-stained smears of sputum can give valuable information about the causal organism and, therefore, aid the choice of antibiotic. Mycological examination of sputum is essential in fungal infections. Examination of suitably stained smears of sputum for mycelial fragments should be performed routinely whenever a fungal pneumonia is suspected (*see* Bronchopulmonary aspergillosis). Methods for culturing viruses, *Legionella pneumophila*, *Mycoplasma pneumoniae*, chlamydiae and coxiellae from sputum are not routinely available.

Anaerobic infections are difficult to confirm bacteriologically because of contamination of sputum with anaerobic bacteria during its passage through the mouth. Tracheal aspiration via the cricothyroid

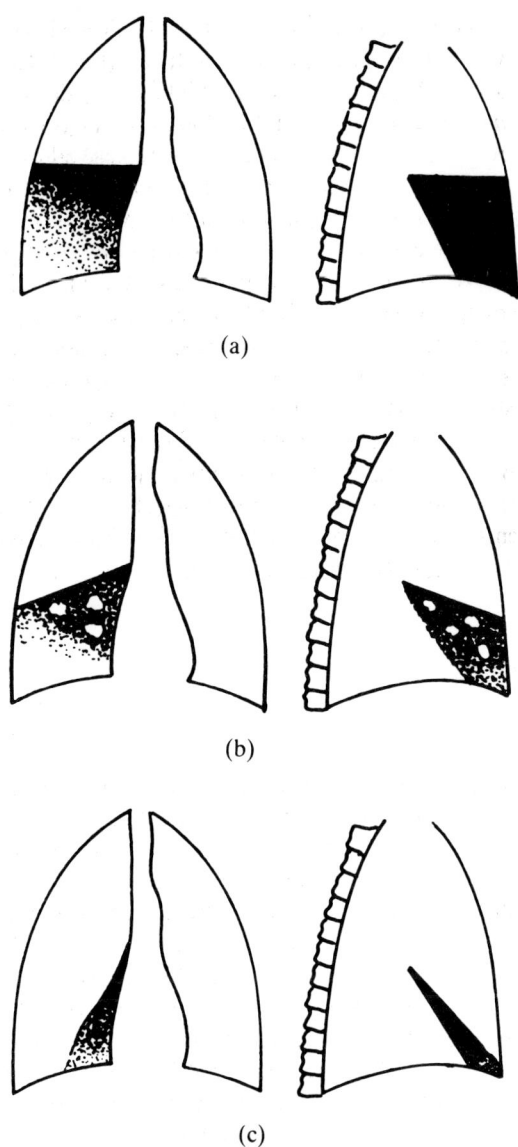

Fig. 7.1 Diagrammatic representation of radiographic features of (a) middle lobe consolidation, (b) middle lobe shrinkage caused by suppurative pneumonia with abscess formation, and (c) middle lobe collapse.

membrane has been advocated to obtain specimens for bacteriological examination for anaerobic organisms.

BLOOD CULTURES

Bacteraemia is common in pneumococcal pneumonia, and septicaemia may be a serious complication of any bacterial pneumonia. Blood for culture should be taken from all ill patients, preferably before antibiotic treatment is started.

SEROLOGY

The diagnosis of viral, coxiellal, chlamydial and mycoplasmal pneumonia can be established retrospectively by the demonstration of a rise in the appropriate antibody titre between two serum specimens, one taken at the beginning of the illness and the other a week later or during the convalescent phase. A fourfold rise in antibody titre is confirmatory evidence of disease. In mycoplasmal pneumonia cold agglutinins are often present in the serum. The demonstration of precipitins, agglutinins and complement-fixing antibodies may be of help in the diagnosis of histoplasmosis. Toxoplasmosis can also be diagnosed by serological tests (Sabin–Feldman dye test). In the much more common pneumococcal infections pneumococcal antigen may be of diagnostic value when detected by counterimmunoelectrophoresis.

WHITE CELL COUNT

The total white cell count is raised in the majority of cases of bacterial pneumonia and the differential count shows a polymorphonuclear leucocytosis. In the majority of cases of non-bacterial pneumonia the total white cell count is usually normal. However, in cases of fulminating bacterial pneumonia the white cell count may be normal or even low in the initial stages.

SKIN TESTS

Useful diagnostic information can be obtained from skin tests in aspergillosis (see Bronchopulmonary aspergillosis), histoplasmosis (intradermal histoplasmin test) and coccidioidomycosis (intradermal coccidioidin test).

LUNG BIOPSY

Fibreoptic bronchoscopy with transbronchial lung biopsy has provided a relatively safe method of obtaining specimens of lung for histological examination even in seriously ill patients. *Pneumocystis carinii* pneumonia cannot be diagnosed satisfactorily without histological examination of infected lung tissue. Bronchial brushings should also be taken but generally are of less value than biopsy or bronchoalveolar lavage.

BRONCHOALVEOLAR LAVAGE

This safe procedure should be performed via the wedged fibreoptic bronchoscope (p. 31) prior to transbronchial lung biopsy or instead of biopsy in thrombocytopenic patients. Cytological examination and culture of the lavage fluid can provide invaluable diagnostic information in patients with obscure pneumonia. This investigation is of particular value in patients who cannot produce sputum.

Differential diagnosis

In the early stages pyrexia may be the only feature and pneumonia may be diagnosed during the investigation of 'pyrexia of unknown origin'. When respiratory symptoms have become established pulmonary infarction often poses a difficult diagnostic problem since pyrexia, breathlessness and pleuritic pain may be the presenting symptoms of both pneumonia and pulmonary infarction. Other causes of pleuritic pain such as tuberculosis and malignant disease must be considered. Cough and purulent sputum may suggest acute bronchitis or an exacerbation of bronchiectasis or chronic bronchitis. Frank haemoptysis is uncommon in pneumonia compared with pulmonary infarction. The association of pleuritic pain and blood-stained purulent sputum suggests suppurative pneumonia, but frank haemoptysis without purulent sputum is more likely to be due to pulmonary infarction. Acute pulmonary tuberculosis may be confused with bacterial pneumonia.

Treatment

General measures

It is extremely important to relieve pleuritic pain adequately. Breathlessness is often largely due to pain. Coughing produces severe distress in the presence of pleuritic pain and is, therefore, consciously suppressed. Only after relief of pain can patients cough efficiently and co-operate with the physiotherapist. Inadequate treatment of pleural pain can result in retention of sputum, bronchial obstruction and pulmonary collapse. Unless there is a contraindication, such as chronic obstructive bronchitis complicated by type II respiratory failure, strong analgesic drugs such as pethidine 50–100 mg intravenously or intramuscularly should be given and repeated as necessary. It is important to co-ordinate the administration of analgesic drugs with physiotherapy. Ideally pethidine should be given an hour before assisted coughing is performed by the physiotherapist or trained nurse so that patient co-operation is not restricted by pain.

Physiotherapy is important in all patients, but overzealous attempts to encourage production of sputum by postural drainage should be avoided in patients with uncomplicated viral pneumonias in which there may be little or no sputum. Postural drainage may be beneficial in patients with bacterial pneumonia and must be performed when pulmonary suppuration and abscess formation have occurred.

Intravenous therapy is necessary in severely ill patients to correct dehydration, to provide a route for the administration of antibiotics and to treat metabolic acidosis and hypotension.

Local treatment of herpes labialis in an attempt to avoid secondary bacterial infection is important. The lesions should be kept dry and, when extensive, acyclovir cream 5% should be applied locally five times daily.

Specific therapy (antibiotics)

In most instances antimicrobial therapy is initiated before a microbiological diagnosis has been established and is subsequently altered if necessary when the aetiological agent has been identified. For practical purposes previously fit subjects developing pneumonia can be assumed to have a pneumococcal infection unless they became ill during a flu epidemic or there is a history suggesting possible exposure to coxiellal, chlamydial or legionella species. It follows that narrow-spectrum chemotherapy is usually appropriate using either penicillin or, to cover 'atypical' organisms, erythromycin. Patients known to be immunosuppressed, or who develop pneumonia while in hospital, may require wider spectrum therapy pending the results of microbiological investigations.

PNEUMOCOCCAL PNEUMONIA

Fortunately very few strains of *Strep. pneumoniae* have acquired resistance to penicillin, and intravenous/intramuscular benzylpenicillin (600 mg twice or thrice daily) is usually recommended. However, oral treatment with ampicillin (250 or 500 mg four times daily) has been shown by clinical trial to be as effective as benzylpenicillin and is a more convenient treatment for both patient and medical staff. In cases of penicillin hypersensitivity erythromycin (250 or 500 mg four times daily) can be used.

STAPHYLOCOCCAL PNEUMONIA

All patients who become rapidly or gravely ill with pneumonia, particularly during an influenza epidemic, should be assumed to have a staphylococcal infection. Intensive antistaphylococcal treatment should be started immediately, even if this means using a combination of several antibiotics, since treatment can be later modified if the causal organism is identified bacteriologically. Staphylococcal infection must be assumed when pneumonia develops in debilitated patients in hospital and also in patients with cystic fibrosis. Treatment with flucloxacillin (250–500 mg four times daily) should be given in patients not known to have penicillin hypersensitivity. In the severely ill parenteral administration should be used initially and benzylpenicillin (600 mg i.v. three times daily) should also be given since it is more effective than flucloxacillin against non-penicillinase producing strains of staphylococci. For patients who are hypersensitive to penicillin, erythromycin (300 or 600 mg i.v. four times daily) or lincomycin (600 mg i.v. twice daily), clindamycin (300 mg i.v. four times daily) or sodium fusidate (580 mg i.v. infusion over 2–4 hours three or four times daily) can be used. In the most gravely ill treatment with gentamicin sulphate (5–6 mg/kg i.v. in divided doses per 24 hours) should also be given if it is uncertain whether the pneumonia is due to *Staph. pyogenes* or one of the Gram-negative bacilli (*see* Treatment of pneumonias caused by Gram-negative bacilli). When improvement in the clinical condition allows, a change from parenteral to oral therapy should be made. Less severely ill patients can be treated with antibiotics by mouth from the outset.

PNEUMONIAS CAUSED BY GRAM-NEGATIVE BACTERIA

Pneumonia caused by Gram-negative bacteria, in particular *Pseudomonas aeruginosa* and proteus organisms, must always be suspected in patients in hospital who are severely debilitated, who are receiving immunosuppressive therapy, or who have a tracheostomy. Gentamicin sulphate and netilimicin sulphate in divided doses of 4–6 mg/kg i.v. per 24 hours are effective drugs for these infections, which seldom respond satisfactorily to ampicillin, tetracycline and co-trimoxazole. Mezlocillin (5 g i.v. infusion three or four times daily) is also useful. Azlocillin (5 g i.v. infusion three times daily) should be used for pseudomonas strains resistant to other antibiotics. For patients with penicillin hypersensitivity, or whenever it is thought likely that a pseudomonas infection is the cause of severe disease, ceftazidime 1–6 g i.v. per 24 hours should be used, with caution, however, because of the possibility of cross-hypersensitivity. *Klebsiella pneumonia* infections should be treated initially with a combination of oral chloramphenicol, 0·5–1 g six-hourly, and i.m. streptomycin sulphate 0·5 or 1 g six-hourly. This drug regimen can be modified if sensitivity tests indicate that the organism is sensitive to co-trimoxazole, a cephalosporin or gentamicin. *In vitro* sensitivity tests suggest that ceftazidime should be an effective treatment of klebsiella infections.

ANAEROBIC INFECTIONS

When infection with anaerobic organisms is suspected, usually because of foul-smelling sputum, treatment with metronidazole (400 mg three times daily) should be given, usually in combination with other anti-bacterial agents. Clindamycin is active against bacteroides strains.

VIRAL PNEUMONIA

Pulmonary infections caused by viruses are not responsive to antibiotic treatment, but if secondary bacterial infection supervenes appropriate treatment should be given.

PNEUMONIA CAUSED BY *MYCOPLASMA PNEUMONIAE*, CHLAMYDIAE, COXIELLAE AND *LEGIONELLA PNEUMOPHILA*

Whenever a diagnosis of mycoplasmal pneumonia, psittacosis or Q fever is suspected treatment with tetracycline (500 mg four times daily) should be given. Doxycycline is possibly more active against *C. burnetii* than other tetracyclines. If there is a contraindication to the use of tetracycline the drug of next choice is erythromycin (500 mg four times daily). In severely ill patients treatment for bacterial pneumonia should also be given initially and an appropriate adjustment of therapy made later according to the results of bacteriological and serological investigations. Legionnaires' disease should be treated with erythromycin 4–6 g daily (i.v. in severely ill) plus rifampicin, 600 mg twice daily.

PNEUMONIA CAUSED BY FUNGI

The most effective treatment for the majority of fungal pneumonias is amphotericin. However, this antibiotic is toxic, particularly to the kidney, and its use must be carefully monitored biochemically and mycologically. Renal toxicity is almost inevitable if a total treatment dose of 5 g is exceeded, but rarely occurs if the cumulative dose can be kept below 2–3 g. The drug is given in a daily dose of 1·0 mg/kg body weight by slow intravenous infusion over a period of six hours. It is usual to start treatment with an initial infusion of 0·25 mg/kg and then to increase the daily dose up to 1·0 mg/kg per 24 hours. Febrile reactions to the drug are common and may be prevented by small doses of hydrocortisone (25–50 mg i.v.) given immediately before, but not with, the amphotericin. The addition of heparin (100 units) to the infusion fluid may decrease thrombophlebitic reactions.

Aspergillus fumigatus pneumonia (invasive pulmonary aspergillosis, p. 128)

Amphotericin is the drug of choice but can be used in combination with flucytosine in some patients. Flucytosine is active against about 75% of aspergillus isolates *in vitro*. A small proportion of aspergillus strains are primarily resistant, and acquired resistance rapidly develops if flucytosine is used as a single treatment. Combination therapy with flucytosine and amphotericin is recommended, since this allows the daily dose of amphotericin to be reduced to 0·5 mg/kg, and emergence of resistance to flucytosine is prevented. Flucytosine should be given orally or intravenously in a dose of 200 mg/kg in four divided doses per 24 hours. Ideally treatment should be monitored by serum levels, and the dose adjusted to maintain a level of between 25 and 80 μg/ml. In cases in which resistance to flucytosine is encountered, amphotericin in full dosage has to be given.

The antifungal imidazoles

These drugs have been found to be generally disappointing in the treatment of fungal pneumonias. Ketoconazole, however, may be of some value in the treatment of coccidioidomycosis and histoplasmosis in a single daily dose of 200–400 mg. This drug should be taken with food and continued for at least a week after the infection appears to have been eradicated.

PNEUMONIA CAUSED BY PROTOZOA

Toxoplasmosis can be treated with a combination of a sulphonamide (1 g four times daily) and pyrimethamine (25 mg daily) for a period of two weeks.

Pneumocystis carinii infections are best treated with 'high-dose' co-trimoxazole (20 mg trimethoprim and 100 mg sulphamethoxazole per kilogram per day in two divided doses i.v.) for two weeks with substitution of oral therapy as soon as is possible. Pentamidine isethionate (4 mg/kg in a single intramuscular daily dose) for 10–14 days has also been recommended but has more side-effects.

Pneumonia in the immunocompromised patient

Pulmonary infection is common in patients receiving immunosuppressive drugs, and in those with diseases resulting in defects of cellular or humoral immune mechanisms. The common pathogenic bacteria are responsible for most infections, but Gram-negative organisms, especially *Pseudomonas aeruginosa,* have become more of a problem in hospital than Gram-positive pathogens, even *Staph. aureus.* In immunocompromised patients unusual organisms, or ones normally considered to be non-pathogenic, may become 'opportunistic' pathogens. Heading the list of opportunists is *Pneumocystis carinii,* followed by fungal infections, especially with candida species and *Aspergillus fumigatus* and viruses such as cytomegalovirus and herpes simplex. *M. tuberculosis* and anaerobic organisms must also be kept in mind, particularly in patients on immunosuppressive drug treatment.

Diagnosis is often very difficult since all the pathogenic organisms and 'opportunists' tend to produce similar clinical and radiological features in immunocompromised patients. Open lung biopsy offers the greatest chance of establishing a diagnosis, but is obviously a high-risk major invasive procedure in such patients. Transbronchial lung biopsy via the fibreoptic bronchoscope should be performed as early as possible when infection with *Pneumocystis carinii* is suspected. Biopsies, bronchial aspirates, bronchoalveolar lavages and brushings should be cultured for bacteria, fungi and viruses, and biopsies, lavages and bronchial brushings examined histologically for *Pneumocystis carinii,* bacteria, fungi and cytomegalovirus inclusion bodies.

Because inappropriate chemotherapy, especially if broad-spectrum, may aggravate fungal infection, wherever possible treatment should be on the basis of a microbiological diagnosis. In practice, however, the cause of the pneumonia is frequently not known when treatment has to be started and hence a combination of drugs chosen to cover a wide range of potential pathogens is given. Mezlocillin, flucloxacillin, gentamicin (or netilmicin) and metronidazole provide a very wide spectrum of activity. Ceftazidime and an antistaphylococcal drug is a good alternative drug combination. If the causative organism is discovered appropriate treatment changes can be made. In other cases when the diagnosis is still in doubt, and there has been no response to the combination of drugs listed above, blind changes or additions to the treatment often have to be made. In individual cases it might seem appropriate to cover the possibility of *Pneumocystis carinii,* tuberculosis, fungal, mycoplasma or legionella infections.

Prognosis

Pneumococcal pneumonia, which at one time was commonly fatal, is now so responsive to treatment that many patients are not admitted to hospital. However, staphylococcal and Gram-negative bacillary pulmonary infections are becoming more common because of immunosuppressive therapy and indiscriminate use of wide-spectrum antibiotics. Prognosis of these infections is often poor unless adequate treatment is started at an early stage. Viral pneumonias and those due to mycoplasma, coxiella, chlamydia and legionella in the main cause mild to moderate disease, but occasionally fulminating fatal infections can occur. Fungal and protozoal pneumonias are uncommon in most parts of the world, but more cases are now being seen, particularly in immunosuppressed patients. In these patients the prognosis is usually bad.

SUMMARY — SPECIAL POINTS OF EMPHASIS

• Pneumonia can be classified anatomically (lobar or lobular) or according to the causative organism (pneumococcal, mycoplasmal).

- The onset of pneumococcal pneumonia is often sudden and dramatic.

- Cough and sputum may be delayed in pneumococcal pneumonia.

- Systemic symptoms are often more pronounced than respiratory symptoms in many non-bacterial pneumonias.

- Complications of pneumonia are:
    Pleural effusion
    Empyema
    Lung abscess
    Collapse
    Type I respiratory failure
    Septicaemia
    Herpes labialis

- Pneumonia in patients with chronic bronchitis often precipitates type II respiratory failure and cor pulmonale.

- Pneumonia can be complicated by thromboembolic disease but pulmonary infarction may be misdiagnosed as pneumonia.

- Consolidation causes decreased chest expansion, dull percussion note, bronchial breathing and whispering pectoriloquy.

- Staphylococcal and Gram-negative bacterial pneumonias most commonly occur in debilitated or immunosuppressed patients.

- Staphylococcal pneumonia is a serious complication of influenza.

- Pneumococcal pneumonia usually heals by resolution without causing lung damage.

- Staphylococcal and Gram-negative bacterial pneumonias usually cause considerable pulmonary damage by suppuration.

- Mental confusion and hyponatraemia are often pronounced in Legionnaires' disease.

- *Pneumocystis carinii,* fungal and viral infections are common in immunocompromised patients, but problems with pathogens such as *Pseudomonas aeruginosa* and *Staph. aureus* are even more common.

- Bacteriological examination of sputum is important, but grossly purulent sputum may not yield a positive culture.

- Pathogenic organisms may be misleadingly cultured from specimens of mucoid sputum. Therefore, do not submit mucoid sputum for bacteriological examination.

• Examination of Gram-stained smears of sputum can give useful therapeutic advice in the very sick patient.

• In general the total white cell count is high in bacterial pneumonias and normal in non-bacterial infections.

• Adequate relief of pleuritic pain is essential.

• *Strep. pneumoniae* is rarely resistant to benzylpenicillin whereas staphylococcal pneumonia almost always is.

• In all gravely ill patients infection with *Staph. aureus* or a Gram-negative organism should be suspected and appropriate treatment started at once.

• Whenever mycoplasmal pneumonia, psittacosis or Q fever is suspected treatment with tetracycline or erythromycin should be given.

Further reading

Pennington J.E. (Ed.) (1983) *Respiratory Infections: Diagnosis and Management.* New York: Raven Press.
Roberts S.O.B., Hay R.J. & Mackenzie D.W.R. (1984) *A Clinician's Guide to Fungal Disease.* New York: Marcel Dekker Inc.
Shanson D.C. (1982) *Microbiology in Clinical Practice.* Bristol: John Wright & Sons Ltd.
Young L.S. (Ed.) (1984) *Pneumocystis carinii Pneumonia.* New York: Marcel Dekker Inc.

Chapter 8
Lung abscess

General considerations

Destruction and cavitation of lung tissue can be the result of a number of pathological processes, but the term lung abscess is usually reserved for suppuration and necrosis caused by bacterial infection. Lung abscess can be caused by:

1 Aspiration pneumonia (secondary pneumonia).
2 Suppurative pneumonia (e.g. staphylococcal).
3 Infection of a pulmonary infarct.

Aspiration pneumonia (secondary pneumonia)

Aspiration pneumonia is caused by the inhalation or 'aspiration' of infected or irritant material from the upper respiratory tract or bronchi to the lungs. This requires:

A source of infected/irritant material

Gastric contents (inhaled vomit), oral sepsis, nasal and sinus infection, bronchial infection (chronic bronchitis and bronchiectasis), infected laryngeal or bronchial tumours.

Interference with the normal coughing mechanism

Unconsciousness, laryngeal palsy, pleuritic, post-operative or traumatic chest pain, extreme debility.

and/or

Interference with tracheobronchial mucociliary clearance

Chronic bronchitis, local and general anaesthesia, bronchial obstruction by secretions, blood clot, foreign body and tumour.

Since these infections occur as consequences of primary disorders (e.g. inhalation of infected material, disordered cough, etc.) the term secondary pneumonia is more appropriate than aspiration pneumonia.

Aspiration pneumonia frequently leads to abscess formation and is the commonest cause of lung abscess. The numerous sources of infection mean that a wide variety of organisms may be responsible for the pulmonary suppuration, some of which are normally of low virulence.

Post-operative 'chest infections' are common and the majority are due to aspiration.

Suppurative pneumonia

Suppurative pneumonia by definition gives rise to pulmonary suppuration, necrosis and abscess formation. This is particularly common in staphylococcal and klebsiella infections when multiple abscesses may form. Pulmonary tuberculosis (p. 246) frequently causes pulmonary destruction. Invasive pulmonary aspergillosis almost always causes pulmonary abscesses. Infection distal to bronchial obstruction by tumour or foreign body may also lead to lung abscess.

Pulmonary infarction

Pulmonary infarction due to septic embolus almost always leads to abscess formation, but this is rare. Infection of simple pulmonary infarcts, however, can produce lung abscesses since infarcted lung tissue provides an ideal nidus for bacterial action to cause suppuration and extensive necrosis.

Rarer causes of lung abscess are traumatic pulmonary injury and extension of suppurative processes from below the diaphragm.

Fundamental points of diagnosis

The diagnosis of lung abscess is usually made radiographically but it must be considered in any patient with pneumonia or pulmonary infarction who suddenly coughs up large amounts of purulent material.

Complications

The complications of lung abscess are:

1 Haemoptysis, which may be massive.
2 Pneumothorax and pyopneumothorax due to destruction of the visceral pleura.

3   Metastatic abscess (e.g. cerebral abscess) due to septic thrombosis of pulmonary veins and systemic embolization.
4   Permanent lung damage which is an inevitable consequence of pulmonary suppuration.

Clinical findings

Symptoms and signs

Patients with lung abscess are usually profoundly ill except in some cases of abscess formation distal to bronchial carcinoma which may cause only slight systemic upset. The onset of disease is usually insidious in the case of aspiration abscess, but is often abrupt and devastating in suppurative pneumonia. As soon as pulmonary necrosis has occurred and there is communication with a bronchus, cough productive of copious amounts of sputum is the most conspicuous feature. The sputum is often foul-smelling and blood-stained. Massive haemoptysis may occur. All the symptoms of pneumonia including pleuritic pain may be present. There is often a high pyrexia which may subside after the abscess has ruptured into a bronchus. Rupture of the abscess into the pleural space with the production of a pyopneumothorax is usually a dramatic event associated with severe pleuritic pain and breathlessness.

The physical findings in the chest are variable. There may be signs of consolidation (p. 92) or signs of pulmonary collapse depending upon whether the bronchus leading to the area of pulmonary suppuration is patent or occluded. Very occasionally 'amphoric' bronchial breath sounds may be heard over large superficial pulmonary abscesses. Often the only detectable clinical abnormality is the presence of inspiratory crepitations. A pleural friction rub may be heard.

Finger clubbing is a feature of lung suppuration and may develop within a couple of weeks after a lung abscess has formed.

Radiological examination

Prior to abscess formation the chest X-ray may show pulmonary shadowing which is usually lobar or segmental, but multiple pulmonary opacities may be seen. After suppuration has occurred and necrotic pulmonary tissue has been coughed up a cavity (Fig. 8.1a) or multiple abscess cavities become evident. Frequently abscess cavities contain fluid levels. There may be radiological evidence of pulmonary collapse and of an underlying bronchial carcinoma (Fig. 8.1b). The X-ray will confirm pneumothorax and the presence of pleural liquid (pyopneumo-thorax) when this serious complication has occurred.

Investigations

Sputum culture may produce a variety of pathogenic organisms. It is common for organisms normally of low virulence to be cultured in aspiration abscesses. In all cases, but particularly when sputum is foul-smelling, anaerobic culture should be performed since anaerobic organisms are frequently present.

The white cell count is usually grossly elevated and the differential white cell count shows a polymorphonuclear leucocytosis.

Other procedures

Bronchoscopic examination is indicated in all patients with evidence of bronchial obstruction. At bronchoscopy any tenacious material which has remained in spite of postural drainage can be removed. Also a diagnosis of bronchial carcinoma can be confirmed when this is the predisposing abnormality. Bronchoscopy is essential when foreign body inhalation is suspected.

Differential diagnosis

The conditions which most often simulate lung abscess are:

Cavitated bronchial carcinoma (Fig. 8.1c)

Often there is no pyrexia or copious sputum production. Radio-graphically the 'abscess cavity' within a carcinoma has an irregular and thick wall compared with a pulmonary abscess, which characteristically has a smooth interior wall and is often relatively thin-walled.

Pulmonary tuberculosis

Cavity formation in tuberculosis is frequent and it is often impossible without bacteriological assistance to differentiate between bacterial suppurative pneumonia and cavitated tuberculosis. After treatment tuberculosis may leave persisting cavities which may radiologically simulate lung abscesses.

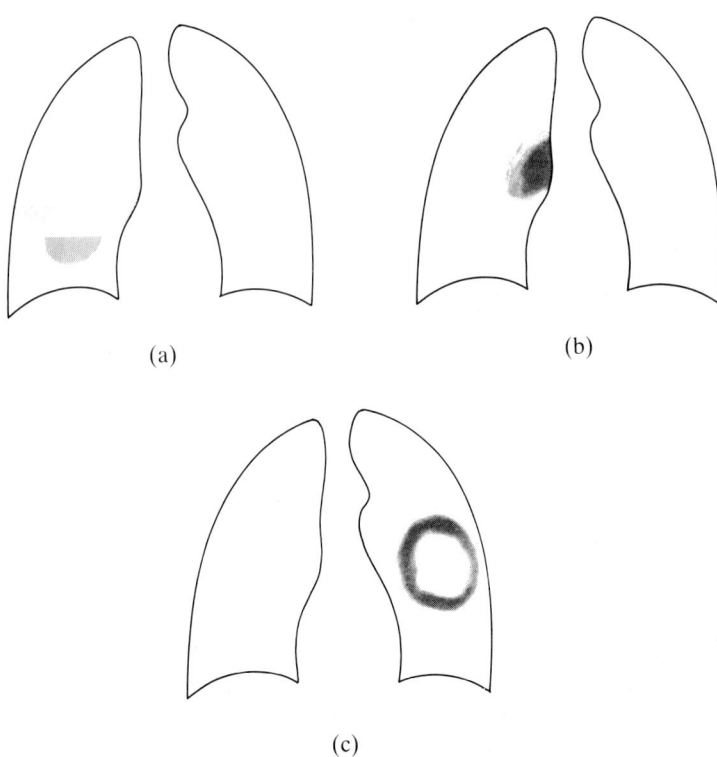

(a)

(b)

(c)

Fig. 8.1 Diagrammatic representation of (a) 'simple' lung abscess within a consolidated middle lobe, (b) lung abscess in a partially collapsed right upper lobe distal to a centrally situated bronchial carcinoma, and (c) irregular cavity within a large peripheral bronchial carcinoma (most which cavitate are squamous).

Hiatus hernia

The X-ray appearances of paraoesophageal hiatus hernia may be mistaken for a lung abscess, particularly in the lateral view. However, these patients usually do not have respiratory symptoms and the diagnosis of hiatus hernia can be confirmed by barium meal examination.

Other conditions which may have to be differentiated from lung abscess are: infected pulmonary bullae, empyema with bronchopleural fistula, cavitated pneumoconiosis, infected bronchogenic cysts, and pulmonary hydatid cysts.

Treatment

Physiotherapy

Postural drainage, combined with chest wall percussion, is necessary to help in the expectoration of inhaled material which may be causing bronchial obstruction, and also to assist drainage of purulent material from abscesses. Physiotherapy with postural drainage must be performed several times every day in the early stages of disease in all patients.

Bronchoscopy

Bronchoscopy may be necessary for the removal of tenacious bronchial secretions and also for diagnostic purposes (*see above*).

Chemotherapy

Choice of antibiotic treatment must be governed by bacteriological examination of sputum. Gram-stained smears can give vital therapeutic advice in the sick patient. The antibiotic treatment of lung abscesses caused by staphylococcal and Gram-negative bacterial infections (p. 103) is the same as for pneumonia but more prolonged courses of treatment are usually necessary. When no pathogenic organisms can be identified ampicillin (500 mg four times daily), flucloxacillin (250–500mg four times daily) and metronidazole (400 mg three times daily) may have to be used in combination. In patients who are penicillin-hypersensitive erythromycin (500 mg four times daily), lincomycin (500 mg three times daily), clindamycin (150–450 mg four times daily) and co-trimoxazole (trimethoprim 80 mg and sulphamethoxazole 400 mg — two tablets twice daily) may be used as alternatives. It is usually necessary to continue antibiotic therapy for a prolonged period of up to six weeks. However, prolonged metronidazole treatment for more than two weeks carries the risk of peripheral neuropathy.

Surgery

Surgical treatment is rarely necessary for simple lung abscess, but when an abscess has developed distal to a bronchial carcinoma or foreign body which cannot be removed bronchoscopically, surgical resection offers the only chance of cure providing there are no contraindications.

Prognosis

The majority of lung abscesses, which are not associated with bronchial carcinoma, respond to treatment if this is energetic and started early. Permanent damage to pulmonary tissue cannot be avoided.

SUMMARY — SPECIAL POINTS OF EMPHASIS

• The commonest causes of lung abscess are aspiration pneumonia, suppurative pneumonia (e.g. staphylococcal) and infection of a pulmonary infarct.

• Aspiration abscesses occur when predisposing abnormalities are present:

    1 A source of infected material.
    2 Interference with the normal defence mechanisms of cough and tracheobronchial mucociliary clearance.

• Organisms causing aspiration lung abscesses may be of low virulence.

• Infection distal to bronchial obstruction by tumour, foreign body, etc. can give rise to lung abscess.

• Examination of Gram-stained smears of sputum can give vital therapeutic advice in the very sick patient.

• Foul-smelling sputum suggests the presence of anaerobic organisms.

• Metronidazole should be used whenever anaerobes have been isolated or are clinically suspected.

• Differentiation between suppurative pneumonia with abscess formation and cavitated tuberculosis may not be possible without bacteriological assistance.

• The diagnosis of lung abscess can usually only be confirmed radiologically.

• Sudden production of copious amounts of purulent sputum by a patient with pneumonia or pulmonary infarction suggests a lung abscess has developed.

- Lung abscess may give rise to massive haemoptysis.

- The physical signs in the chest may be those of consolidation, collapse or merely the presence of inspiratory crepitations. 'Amphoric' bronchial breath sounds are rarely heard.

- Finger clubbing may develop within 2-3 weeks.

- Bronchoscopy is often necessary therapeutically for the removal of material causing bronchial obstruction and also for diagnostic purposes when an underlying carcinoma is suspected.

- Cavitation of a bronchial carcinoma often simulates lung abscess.

- Postural drainage and chest wall percussion is an important part of treatment in all cases.

- Antibiotic treatment has to be given for a prolonged period.

- If there is doubt, it is advisable to cover the possibility of staphylococcal infection.

Further reading

Pennington J.E. (Ed.) (1983) *Respiratory Infections: Diagnosis and Management.* New York: Raven Press.
Roberts S.O.B., Hay R.J. & Mackenzie D.W.R. (1984) *A Clinician's Guide to Fungal Disease.* New York: Marcel Dekker Inc.
Shanson D.C. (1982) *Microbiology in Clnical Practice.* Bristol: John Wright & Sons Ltd.

Chapter 9
Bronchopulmonary aspergillosis

General considerations

Aspergillosis in its various forms is by far the most common respiratory fungal disorder in Britain and countries with similar climatic conditions. Aspergillus species are soil organisms and their spores are almost constantly present in the atmosphere. The inhalation of fungal spores rarely gives rise to disease in normal individuals but can lead to a number of problems in patients with pre-existent respiratory disorders. Most cases of aspergillosis are caused by *A. fumigatus*, but other members of the genus (*A. clavatus, A. flavus, A. niger* and *A. terreus*) occasionally cause disease. Bronchopulmonary aspergillosis can be classified into five main groups:

1 Allergic asthma.
2 Allergic bronchopulmonary aspergillosis (asthmatic pulmonary eosinophilia).
3 Extrinsic allergic alveolitis.
4 Intracavitary aspergilloma.
5 Invasive pulmonary aspergillosis.

Dissemination to involve all tissues of the body is a rare but often fatal complication which is usually associated with immunosuppressive drug therapy.

Fundamental points of diagnosis

Although the various clinical types of aspergillosis have different clinical pictures the investigations necessary to establish a diagnosis are similar:

1 Mycological examination of sputum.
2 Demonstration of antibodies in the serum.
3 Demonstration of skin hypersensitivity to extracts of the fungus.

Interpretation of the results of sputum culture can be difficult since a positive culture may simply be due to the inhalation of fungal spores or contamination of culture plates in a laboratory. A growth of *A. fumigatus* from sputum often is not indicative of disease but all heavy growths should be regarded with enough suspicion to stimulate further investigation. The presence of fungal hyphae on microscopic examination of smears of sputum or bronchial aspirates is diagnostic, since this indicates fungal growth within the respiratory tract. Fungal hyphae are usually abundant in bronchial casts produced by patients with allergic bronchopulmonary aspergillosis. A negative sputum culture does not exclude aspergillosis, since the production of fungus in the sputum varies considerably from day to day in some types of this disease.

Precipitating antibodies are present in the serum of most patients with aspergillosis, but antibody formation can be suppressed by systemic corticosteroid therapy. Techniques involving antibody fluorescence and radioimmunoassay may be used to demonstrate fungal antibodies in blood.

Skin tests performed with extracts of the fungus can show an immediate and/or late reaction in different types of aspergillosis. Skin hypersensitivity to *A. fumigatus* is not a feature of all types of bronchopulmonary aspergillosis.

The fundamental points of diagnosis of the different forms of bronchopulmonary aspergillosis are summarized in Table 9.1

ALLERGIC ASTHMA

Hypersensitivity to *A. fumigatus* can be demonstrated in some patients with chronic asthma and the fungus may be isolated from sputum. It is possible that the development of hypersensitivity to *A. fumigatus* in patients with chronic asthma is responsible for worsening of symptoms, but this is difficult to establish with certainty. It is likely that the course of asthma is not radically altered in these patients, unless asthmatic pulmonary eosinophilia develops.

ALLERGIC BRONCHOPULMONARY ASPERGILLOSIS

General considerations

Pulmonary radiographic shadowing accompanied by a high peripheral blood eosinophil count (*see* Pulmonary eosinophilia) is a serious but uncommon complication of asthma which radically alters the prognosis. The majority of cases of allergic bronchopulmonary aspergillosis are due to colonization of the bronchi with *A. fumigatus* and the development of hypersensitivity reactions to the presence of this fungus.

Fundamental points of diagnosis

The radiographic abnormalities are of two types (*see below*). The diagnosis should always be considered in an asthmatic patient with an

Table 9.1 Diagnosis of different forms of bronchopulmonary aspergillosis.

Type	Sputum	Serological tests	Eosinophils	Skin tests	X-ray	Comment
Allergic asthma	+/- micro +/- culture	May be positive	Usually raised	+	Normal	Clinical effects of fungus difficult to assess
Asthmatic pulmonary eosinophilia	+ micro + culture	Positive	High	+	Fleeting pulmonary shadows often segmental	Leads to bronchiectasis
Extrinsic allergic alveolitis	+ micro + culture	Positive	Normal	Usually negative	Diffuse patchy and reticular shadows	If not treated leads to diffuse pulmonary fibrosis
Intracavitary aspergilloma	+ micro + culture	Positive	Normal	Usually negative	Fungus ball within cavity	Usually benign
Invasive pulmonary aspergillosis	+ micro + culture	Positive (unless on corticosteroids)	Normal	Usually negative	Gross pulmonary destruction	Often fatal

high peripheral blood eosinophil count and an X-ray abnormality. Fungal hyphae are visible in stained smears of sputum and are usually abundant in bronchial casts. *A. fumigatus* is cultured from sputum but the amount of fungus produced in the sputum varies considerably from day to day. A single negative culture for *A. fumigatus* does not exclude the disease. Skin tests with extracts of *A. fumigatus* produce a positive immediate reaction in all cases and a late (positive at six hours) reaction in a proportion of patients. Precipitating antibodies to *A. fumigatus* are present in the serum of all patients.

Complications

Bronchiectasis at the site of the radiographic pulmonary shadows is the major complication. This is a frequent and serious complication of untreated lobar or segmental collapse. The bronchiectasis in asthmatic pulmonary eosinophilia is often proximal and tends to affect the upper more than the lower lobes.

Clinical findings

Symptoms and signs

Episodes of allergic bronchopulmonary aspergillosis classically are associated with mild fever and an exacerbation of symptoms of asthma. However, it is not uncommon for the pulmonary abnormalities to develop without clinical deterioration of asthma and only be detected by routine X-ray examination. Bronchial casts are frequently produced in the sputum, but these may not be conspicuous at an early stage since they are often coughed up only during the recovery phase. Occlusion of a major bronchus may cause breathlessness without wheeze, and produce the clinical signs of lobar collapse. In the absence of major pulmonary collapse the findings are those of asthma and bronchiectasis. In patients in whom repeated episodes of pulmonary eosinophilia have caused widespread bronchiectasis the symptoms and signs of this disease dominate the clinical picture.

Radiological examination

Chest X-ray abnormalities, which are often described as fleeting and recurrent, are of four main types (Fig. 9.1):

1   Areas of pulmonary collapse (collapse/consolidation).

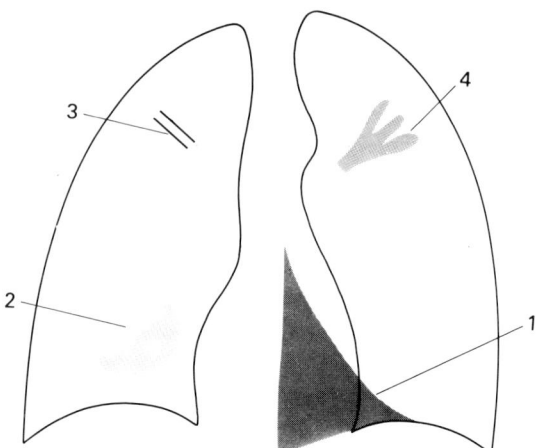

Fig. 9.1 Diagrammatic representation of the radiographic abnormalities seen in allergic bronchopulmonary aspergillosis. (1) Collapse of a lobe or segment (left lower lobe collapse seen 'behind' the cardiac shadow). (2) Diffuse pulmonary shadowing (shown in the right middle and lower zones). (3) 'Tramline' shadows (right upper zone). (4) 'Glove' shadow (left upper zone).

2 Peripheral pulmonary shadows of variable extent and appearance.
3 Thickened bronchial walls appearing on X-rays as 'tram-line' shadows.
4 Finger-like shadows caused by mucoid impaction within dilated bronchi.

Pulmonary collapse (collapse/consolidation)

This may be segmental, lobar or even total lung collapse. The upper lobes are more frequently involved than the lower. These radiological abnormalities are due to the occlusion of large bronchi by mucous plugs and are similar to the X-ray changes produced by bronchial obstruction of any cause, e.g. bronchial carcinoma.

Peripheral pulmonary shadows

These can be of infinite variety and may be multiple and bilateral. Homogeneous pulmonary shadows are most frequent, but pulmonary mottling and peribronchial infiltrations are not uncommon.

Tram-line shadows and those of mucoid impaction are not as common as those described above and are often difficult to interpret.

Investigations

Blood

A high eosinophil count accompanies each episode. Precipitating antibodies to *A. fumigatus* are present in the serum of the vast majority of patients but negative results may be obtained between episodes.

Skin tests

A positive immediate prick skin test reaction to an extract of *A. fumigatus* is found in all cases. A negative skin reaction can be used as evidence that the pulmonary eosinophilia is not associated with hypersensitivity to this fungus. In some patients a late skin reaction can be observed at six hours.

Mycological examination

Fungal hyphae can be demonstrated in the sputum in all patients at some stage of the disease. However, the amount of fungus present in the sputum in asthmatic pulmonary eosinophilia is much more variable than in any other type of bronchopulmonary aspergillosis. When bronchial obstruction has occurred during an episode there may be no fungus in the sputum, but large amounts may be present during the recovery phase when bronchial casts are expectorated. Mucous plugs removed at bronchoscopy usually have abundant mycelial elements visible on microscopy and yield heavy growths of fungus on culture. The absence of fungus in a mucous plug in contrast with sputum is strong evidence that the disease is not due to *A. fumigatus*.

Bronchoscopy

Bronchoscopy is necessary in many cases with radiological evidence of pulmonary collapse for both diagnostic and therapeutic reasons. Other causes of collapse (e.g. bronchial carcinoma) can only be excluded by bronchoscopy, which also allows the removal of mucous plugs. Following bronchoscopic removal of casts radiographic evidence of collapse can be expected to disappear within a few hours.

Differential diagnosis

The X-ray changes in asthmatic pulmonary eosinophilia are so varied that all pulmonary disease associated with a radiological pulmonary abnormality can be simulated. However, bronchial carcinoma, pneumonia and tuberculosis are the most important diseases involved in the differential diagnosis.

Treatment

The efficacy of treatment must be assessed by its ability to prevent bronchiectasis which still complicates many cases. All patients must have optimal treatment of their asthma. It is now agreed that oral corticosteroid therapy with prednisolone in a dose of 20–40 mg daily is necessary for the treatment of episodes of asthmatic pulmonary eosinophilia. Patients with rapidly recurring disease should have maintenance therapy with prednisolone in a daily dose of 10 mg initially, reducing as indicated to find the optimum minimal dose for each individual patient. Inhaled corticosteroid therapy does not prevent episodes of asthmatic pulmonary eosinophilia and is only useful for the treatment of the asthmatic symptoms. The value of high-dose inhaled corticosteroids (e.g. beclomethasone dipropionate or budesonide 1.5 mg or more daily) has not been assessed.

Bronchoscopy is necessary in the treatment of pulmonary collapse whenever high-dose prednisolone therapy, together with vigorous physiotherapy and treatment with bronchodilator drugs, has failed to achieve reaeration of pulmonary tissue within a few days.

Irradication of fungal colonization using drugs by inhalation (e.g. natamycin) is only temporarily effective and is rarely indicated. The presently available systemically administered antifungal agents are probably of no value in the treatment of this condition.

Bronchiectasis should be treated by physiotherapy and antibiotics as necessary (p. 52).

Prognosis

The prognosis of asthma complicated by pulmonary eosinophilia is very much worse than that of uncomplicated asthma because of the development of bronchiectasis. The prognosis in individual cases depends upon the frequency of episodes of pulmonary eosinophilia and their response to treatment. Early death from cor pulmonale and type II respiratory failure occurs in patients who develop extensive bronchiectasis.

EXTRINSIC ALLERGIC ALVEOLITIS

Extrinsic allergic alveolitis (*see* p. 197) has been shown to result from massive exposure of maltworkers to *A. clavatus*. The clinical features of this disease are similar to those of other types of extrinsic allergic alveolitis (e.g. farmer's lung). The diagnosis is made from the occupational history and the demonstration of serum precipitins to *A. clavatus*. In doubtful cases provocation tests may be of value.

INTRACAVITARY ASPERGILLOMA

General considerations

An aspergilloma, or ball of aspergillus fungus (Fig. 9.2), can form in any area of damaged pulmonary tissue in which there is a persistent abnormal space. The most common cause of such pulmonary damage is tuberculosis, but aspergillomas can develop in abscess cavities, bronchiectatic spaces and cavitated tumours. Aspergillomas do not occur in healthy lungs. Most, but not all, are caused by *A. fumigatus*.

Fundamental points of diagnosis

1 Radiological demonstration of a fungus ball (*see below*).
2 Serum precipitins to *A. fumigatus*.

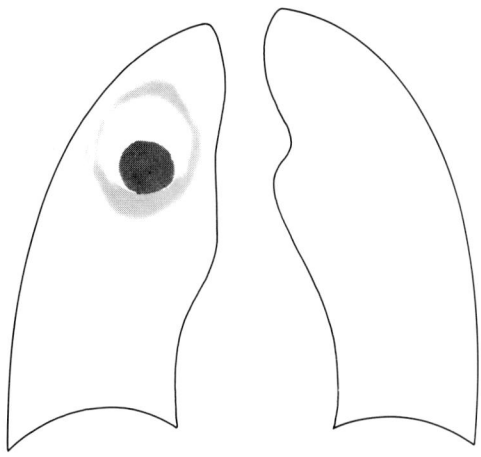

Fig. 9.2 Diagrammatic representation of a fungus ball within a cavity in the right upper zone.

3   Haemoptysis is the most common symptom but many aspergillomas are asymptomatic.

Complications

The most serious complications are:

1   Recurrent haemoptysis, which may be massive and fatal.
2   General debility, weight loss.
3   Invasion of surrounding lung tissue by *A. fumigatus* — invasive pulmonary aspergillosis (p. 128). This is a rare but grave complication and may be induced by immunosuppressive drug therapy.

Clinical findings

Symptoms and signs

Many aspergillomas are asymptomatic and are diagnosed by routine chest X-ray. The most common symptom is haemoptysis, which is usually recurrent and may be massive and fatal. Systemic symptoms are not common, but general debility and weight loss occurs in a few patients. There are no specific clinical findings. Most patients have the clinical findings of the underlying disease, e.g. inactive pulmonary tuberculosis, bronchiectasis.

Radiological examination

The chest X-ray is the single most important investigation in the diagnosis of aspergilloma. X-rays taken prior to the development of the fungus ball may show a cavity or cystic space. The aspergilloma appears as a solid opacity within the cavity and is usually spherical and may appear to fill the cavity totally. Tomography may be necessary to show the aspergilloma to be separated from the walls of the cavity by an air space or 'halo'.

Investigations

Sputum

Sputum of patients with an aspergilloma consistently shows the presence of hyphae on microscopy and produces a positive culture. Failure to demonstrate *A. fumigatus* in the sputum virtually excludes the diagnosis.

Blood

The vast majority of patients with an aspergilloma have precipitating antibodies to the offending fungus (usually *A. fumigatus*) in the serum. If the aspergilloma has developed while the patient has been treated with systemic corticosteroids serum precipitins may be absent.

Skin tests

Approximately one-third of patients exhibit skin hypersensitivity to *A. fumigatus*.

Differential diagnosis

The chest X-ray often suggests a peripheral tumour and this diagnosis may appear to be supported by the history since haemoptysis is the most frequent symptom. Haemoptysis, however, may also suggest a recurrence of tuberculosis.

Treatment

Most aspergillomas do not require specific therapy. When recurrent haemoptysis and general ill health are features of this disease surgical removal of the fungus ball is the only treatment that offers permanent cure. Unfortunately, most patients, because of the underlying pathology, are not suitable candidates for thoracotomy. Local incision of the chest wall and removal of the aspergilloma without attempts to remove the lung cavity have occasionally been performed with success. However, recurrence is common after this procedure. Drug therapy is generally unsatisfactory. Long-term treatment with oral corticosteroids and antibiotics should be avoided because of the risk of inducing invasive pulmonary aspergillosis.

Prognosis

In most patients the development of an aspergilloma does not significantly alter the prognosis, which is often poor because of the underlying pulmonary damage. Haemoptysis may be trivial and recurrent over many years but must be taken seriously because of the possibility of massive pulmonary bleeding. General ill health and weight loss associated with an aspergilloma usually mean a poor prognosis unless surgical removal of the aspergilloma is possible.

INVASIVE PULMONARY ASPERGILLOSIS

Invasion of previously healthy lung tissue by *A. fumigatus* is uncommon. It is usually induced by immunosuppressive therapy and prolonged treatment with wide-spectrum antibiotics. It causes massive pulmonary destruction and carries a very poor prognosis. The course of disease is usually relentless with the formation of multiple abscesses and the production of copious amounts of blood-stained sputum. This rare disease usually occurs in patients with known bronchopulmonary aspergillosis and should be suspected in any such patient who develops a suppurative pneumonia unresponsive to conventional treatment. Fungal elements are present in abundance in the sputum and serum precipitins can be demonstrated in all patients not receiving massive doses of corticosteroids. If diagnosed at an early stage treatment with amphotericin in combination with flucytosine can be successful (*see* p. 105).

SUMMARY — SPECIAL POINTS OF EMPHASIS

• *A. fumigatus* is the most common cause of bronchopulmonary fungal disease in Britain.

• The most important clinical types of bronchopulmonary aspergillosis are asthmatic pulmonary eosinophilia and intracavitary aspergilloma.

• The microscopical visualization of hyphae in sputum indicates fungal colonization of some part of the respiratory tract and is always of diagnostic significance.

• Allergic bronchopulmonary aspergillosis can cause widespread bronchiectasis.

• Oral corticosteroid therapy and optimal treatment with bronchodilators is indicated in most cases of asthmatic pulmonary eosinophilia due to *A. fumigatus*.

• Aspergilloma is the result of colonization by fungus of bronchial cavities caused by previous disease.

• The majority of patients who develop an aspergilloma do not have symptoms.

• The most common symptom of aspergilloma is haemoptysis.

• Necrotizing pulmonary aspergillosis is uncommon but can be induced by immunosuppressive therapy and is often fatal.

• Invasive pulmonary aspergillosis is usually induced by immunosuppressive treatment of patients already known to have a form of bronchopulmonary aspergillosis but should be suspected in all cases of 'suppurative pneumonia'.

Further reading

Conant N.F., Smith D.T., Baker R.D. & Gallaway J.L. (1971) *Manual of Clinical Mycology*. Philadelphia: W.B. Saunders & Co.

Emmons C.W., Binford C.H. & Utz J.P. (1977) *Medical Mycology,* 3rd Edition. Philadelphia: Lea & Febiger.

Pennington J.E. (Ed.) (1983) *Respiratory Infections: Diagnosis and Management.* New York: Raven Press.

Roberts S.O.B., Hay R.J. & Mackenzie D.W.R. (1984) *A Clinician's Guide to Fungal Disease.* New York: Marcel Dekker Inc.

Wilson J.W. & Plunkett Orda A. (1965) *The Fungus Diseases of Man.* Berkeley: University of California Press.

Chapter 10
Tumours of the lungs

INTRODUCTION

Trachea	Primary malignant	— rare
	Secondary malignant	— rare
	Benign	— rare

Bronchi	Primary malignant	— very common
	Secondary malignant	— rare
	Benign	— uncommon

Lungs	Primary malignant	— uncommon
	Secondary malignant	— common
	Benign	— rare

Tumours of the trachea are very rare. Benign or low-malignancy adenomas of the trachea are occasionally found, usually at its lower end, which is more often involved by direct extension of tumours arising in the main bronchi. Partial obstruction of the trachea by tumour usually presents with stridor and breathlessness which may simulate asthma. The trachea may be compressed by tumour masses in the mediastinum but metastatic deposits in the tracheal wall are extremely rare.

Carcinoma of the bronchus is a very common malignant lesion. Secondary malignant deposits in the bronchi are uncommon, but bronchi may be involved by extension of metastases in the lung. Bronchial adenoma is rare compared with carcinoma.

Primary malignant tumours of the lung (bronchioloalveolar cell carcinoma) are rare compared with bronchial carcinoma but blood-borne metastatic deposits from primary sites elsewhere in the body are common. Benign pulmonary tumours are extremely rare.

CARCINOMA OF THE BRONCHUS

General considerations

Carcinoma of the bronchus is the commonest malignant neoplasm encountered in clinical practice in the United Kingdom and the mortality from this tumour has steadily risen during the last three decades. It is somewhat more common in males and occurs mainly in the middle-aged and elderly. There is a definite causal relationship with cigarette smoking, and pipe and cigar smokers who inhale have a higher incidence than non-smokers. Atmospheric pollution plays a much less important role, but urban dwellers have a slightly higher incidence than people living in rural areas. The industrial hazards which have been shown to cause carcinoma of the bronchus include asbestos, pitchblende, haematite, chromate, nickel and arsenic. However, the major association is with cigarette smoking.

Pathological types of malignant primary lung tumours

Squamous carcinoma	35%
Undifferentiated small cell carcinoma	24%
Adenocarcinoma	21%
Undifferentiated large cell carcinoma	19%
Others	1%

Bronchioloalveolar cell
   carcinoma
Carcinoid tumours   } bronchial adenoma
Adenoid cystic carcinoma }

Fundamental points of diagnosis and complications

Bronchial carcinoma may present because of:

Local effects of tumour in the bronchus

Cough
Haemoptysis
Breathlessness (or stridor)
Infection beyond tumour obstruction of the bronchus.

Spread to the pleura and chest wall

Pleural pain
Chest wall pain
Pleural effusion.

Spread to mediastinum

Hoarseness and bovine cough
Superior vena caval obstruction (Fig. 10.1)

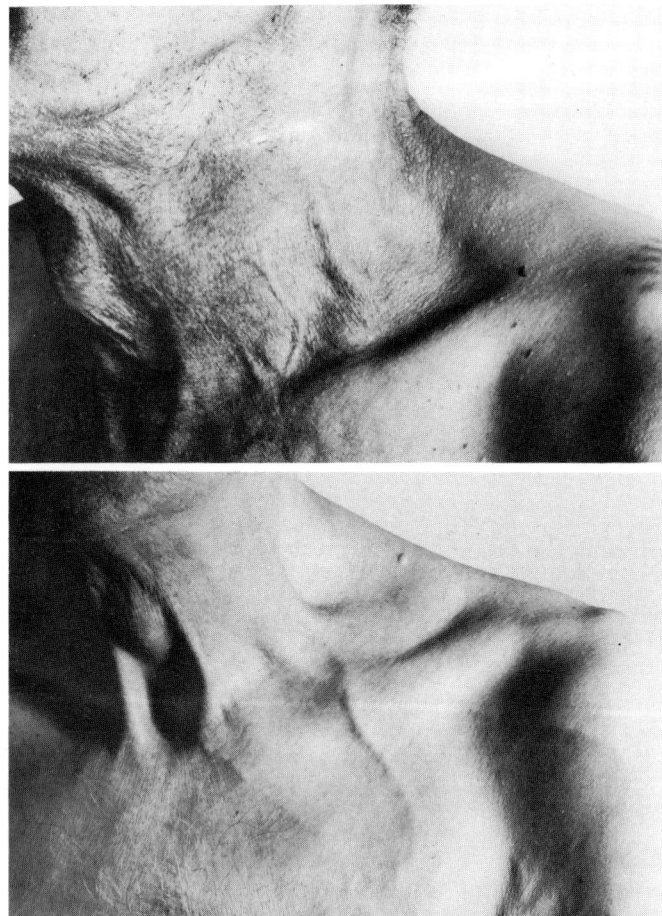

Fig. 10.1 Superior vena caval obstruction: engorged neck veins and anastomotic veins on anterior chest wall.

Dysphagia
Phrenic nerve paralysis
Pancoast tumour.

Lymphatic spread to the neck

Enlarged cervical glands.

Distant blood-borne metastatic spread

Cerebral symptoms
Bone pain
Hepatomegaly.

Non-metastatic syndromes

Endocrine
Neurological.

Non-specific symptoms of ill-health

Weight loss
Lethargy.

Routine X-ray detection

Symptomless lesion.

The symptoms in any particular patient will largely depend upon the presence or absence of these various complications, and it is important to appreciate that severe metastatic or non-metastatic complications may arise in the absence of any local features of disease.

Clinical symptoms

Symptoms due to tumour in a bronchus

Cough

Cough is the commonest early symptom in 'uncomplicated' carcinoma. However, since most patients also have a 'smoker's cough' they often delay seeking medical advice. Many present in late spring or early summer because a 'winter cough' has not cleared up with the onset of good weather. Usually the cough is entirely non-specific, but bronchial carcinoma is by far the most frequent cause of left recurrent laryngeal nerve paralysis. Sometimes such patients have noticed that cough has become less efficient (bovine cough) but their main complaint is usually hoarseness.

Haemoptysis

Haemoptysis is a commom symptom of carcinomas arising in major bronchi (central tumours), but is less common in peripheral tumours. The usual description is blood streaking of sputum, particularly in the mornings, and is due to ulceration of the tumour surface, whereby sputum passing over the lesion becomes streaked with blood. Scanty haemoptysis of this type may be continuous or intermittent and many patients do not seek medical advice for prolonged periods because of the apparently trivial nature of this complaint. Centrally situated tumours can invade large pulmonary vessels and cause massive haemoptysis, which is often fatal.

Breathlessness and stridor

Breathlessness is usually caused by tumour obstructing large bronchi. Peripheral tumours are associated with dyspnoea only when they are so huge as to interfere with pulmonary function, or when spread to sub-carinal glands causes compression of the central large airways, or when complicated by a massive pleural effusion. Shortness of breath is the major complaint in lymphatic carcinomatosis (p. 144).

There is usually clinical evidence of collapse (complete bronchial obstruction) or obstructive emphysema (occlusion on expiration but not on inspiration). Narrowing of a large bronchus may be noticed by the patient as a 'wheeze' in one place or by the clinician as a 'fixed rhonchus' unaltered by coughing. Stridor is produced by partial occlusion of the main bronchi or lower end of the trachea, and although it may be obvious clinically the patient's complaint is usually of breathlessness and wheeze.

Infection distal to bronchial carcinoma

Obstruction of the bronchus often leads to distal infection because of interference with bronchial drainage. This can present clinically as:

1   Pneumonia which is slow to respond to treatment.
2   Recurrent episodes of pneumonia in the same site.
3   Lung abscess distal to a carcinoma (necrosis and cavitation of a tumour can also simulate lung abscess).

Sputum in bronchial carcinoma

Although the tumour itself does not cause sputum production many patients are smokers with chronic bronchitis and therefore have sputum. Infected sputum is found when partial bronchial obstruction leads to distal infection, but not when a tumour completely occludes the affected bronchus.

Spread to pleura

Symptoms produced by spread to the pleura are often the presenting features. Involvement of the pleura almost always indicates the tumour is inoperable, and may cause:

1   Pleural effusion.
2   Pleuritic pain.
3   Chest wall pain when the tumour has spread beyond the parietal pleura.

Pleural effusion and pleuritic pain may be caused by infection distal to the carcinoma and hence are not always evidence that the tumour is inoperable. Full investigation of the effusion is, therefore, imperative to determine the cause — malignant or infective. Malignant effusions tend to be blood-stained and rapidly recur after aspiration.

Constant chest wall pain unrelated to breathing suggests invasion of the chest wall.

Spread to mediastinum

Mediastinal structures are involved by spread to mediastinal lymph glands (common) or by direct extension of the tumour mass (less common). Evidence of mediastinal spread almost invariably means the tumour is inoperable. Tumour invasion of the mediastinum can present as:

1   Left recurrent laryngeal nerve palsy.
2   Superior vena caval obstruction.
3   Dysphagia.
4   Phrenic nerve paralysis.
5   Apical tumours involving brachial plexus and sympathetic ganglia ('Pancoast' tumours).

Pancoast's syndrome (first described by Hare in 1838 and, therefore, sometimes referred to as Hare–Pancoast syndrome) is characterized by pain in the shoulder and arm plus ipsilateral Horner's syndrome. The pain, which is often associated with numbness and tingling, usually starts in the shoulder then extends down the inside of the arm to the elbow and later down the ulnar side of the forearm to include the 4th and 5th fingers. Subsequently weakness and wasting of the hand occur. Pain is caused by compression and/or infiltration of the brachial plexus. Horner's syndrome is characterized by a decreased palpebral fissure, ipsilateral anhydrosis, enophthalmos and constriction of the pupil and is caused by involvement of the sympathetic chain and stellate ganglion on or near the neck of the first rib. Pancoast's syndrome is not a pathological entity and can be caused by any lesion arising in the thoracic inlet. Primary bronchial carcinoma is by far the most common cause; over 50% are squamous tumours and the remainder are mainly large cell and adenocarcinomas. Other malignant lesions such as myeloma, mesothelioma and Hodgkin's disease can cause this syndrome and nonmalignant causes such as pulmonary tuberculosis, hydatid disease and osteomyelitis with an associated abscess have been described.

Pancoast tumours often also invade adjacent ribs (usually the first) and vertebrae. Extension of tumour through an intervertebral foramen may cause spinal cord compression.

Lymphatic spread

Lymphatic spread of lung cancer occurs initially to ipsilateral hilar nodes, then to mediastinal and subsequently to scalene and coeliac nodes. The group of nodes around the trachea and main bronchi is accessible to mediastinoscopy (p. 148). Left upper lobe cancers first spread to glands anterior to the aortic arch, and a more reliable way of detecting lymphatic metastatic spread in this site is anterior mediastinotomy. Careful examination of the neck for enlarged glands, especially in the scalene areas, is perhaps the most important part of the examination of a patient with bronchial carcinoma or suspected to have this disease.

Distant blood-borne metastatic spread

Bronchial carcinomas, particularly anaplastic tumours, often metastasize widely at an early stage. Hence, evidence of disease in any organ or body tissue can be the first evidence of a primary carcinoma in the bronchus. Metastatic spread to liver, bone, skin and brain is particularly common.

Non-metastatic syndromes

The cells of the bronchial tumour can produce biologically active hormone-like substances (usually peptides). The exact incidence of these abnormalities is not known. However, clinical presentation with symptoms of a non-metastatic syndrome alone is unusual. These syndromes can be conveniently divided into two groups, endocrine and neuromuscular. Most of the endocrine syndromes are associated with small cell tumours. Hypercalcaemia is, however, more common in squamous carcinoma.

NON-METASTATIC ENDOCRINE SYNDROMES

Hyponatraemia (inappropriate antidiuretic hormone secretion)

Symptoms not always present but can cause drowsiness, lethargy and disorientation.

Ectopic ACTH syndrome

The full clinical picture of Cushing's syndrome is rare but oedema, muscle weakness, skin pigmentation and hypertension can occur. A common biochemical finding is hypokalaemic alkalosis.

Hypercalcaemia

This can be a manifestation of a non-metastatic syndrome due to secretion of a parathormone-like substance, but is more often due to bony metastatic deposits. Clinical effects can be malaise, thirst, polyuria, nausea, drowsiness, confusion and coma.

Other less common non-metastatic endocrine syndromes

1 Carcinoid syndrome (more often associated with adenoma than carcinoma).
2 Hyperthyroidism.
3 Hypoglycaemia.
4 Gynaecomastia (usually associated with hypertrophic pulmonary osteoarthropathy [HPOA] but can occur on its own).
5 Red cell aplasia.
6 Skin pigmentation (in absence of other manifestations of ectopic ACTH secretion).

NON-METASTATIC 'NEUROMUSCULAR' SYNDROMES

These conditions are unrelated to metastatic tumour dissemination and their pathogenesis is unknown. Florid forms are uncommon but they may result in the patient's referral to a neurologist. The syndromes include:

1 *Neuropathies* (sensory, motor and mixed peripheral neuropathies have all been well documented).
2 *Cerebellar degeneration.*
3 *Mental abnormalities* such as progressive dementia.
4 *Autonomic dysfunction* causing postural hypotension.
5 *Myopathies.*
6 *Myopathic-myasthenic syndrome* (Eaton–Lambert syndrome).
7 *Motor neurone-like disease.*

OTHER NON-METASTATIC SYNDROMES

Hypertrophic pulmonary osteoarthropathy (HPOA)

It is customary to describe this syndrome separately from the non-metastatic syndromes. It is more frequent than the syndromes listed above and it is a fairly common presentation of this disease. The characteristic symptom is pain, which may be severe, usually in the wrists and ankles but also in the knees and shins. The distal parts of the long bones of the wrists and ankles may be exquisitely tender to touch and pitting oedema is often present over the anterior aspect of the shin. Finger clubbing, usually marked, is present in nearly all cases and gynaecomastia may also be part of the syndrome. Blood flow to the affected limbs and bones is increased. Pathologically there is periosteal new bone formation, which can be readily detected radiographically. The cause of HPOA is unknown. Symptoms can be relieved by removal of the tumour, vagotomy or even thoracotomy without any other operative procedure. HPOA is most frequently associated with bronchial carcinoma but occurs with other tumours such as pleural fibroma and renal carcinoma. It has also been described in association with cystic fibrosis.

Finger clubbing

Finger clubbing in any adult patient, especially a smoker, should raise the possibility of bronchial carcinoma. Clubbing could be regarded as the most common non-metastatic manifestation.

Non-specific symptoms of ill-health

Carcinoma of the bronchus may never produce specific symptoms and hence present at a late stage with general debility, anorexia, and extreme weight loss and wasting.

Chest X-ray abnormality in symptomless patient

Bronchial carcinoma is often detected as an X-ray abnormality picked up on routine screening. Unfortunately, the prognosis of patients diagnosed in this way is little better than that of the patient with symptoms.

Clinical findings

Physical signs in the chest

Examination is usually normal unless significant bronchial obstruction has been produced, or spread to the pleura has taken place.

Abnormal physical findings due to bronchial obstruction

Complete bronchial obstruction. Signs of collapse of a lobe or lung — segmental collapse is often clinically undetectable.

Partial bronchial obstruction. May cause:

1 A 'fixed' or 'localized' rhonchus over the site of bronchial narrowing which is not abolished by coughing.
2 Reduced air entry to the area of lung distal to the partial bronchial obstruction.
3 'Obstructive emphysema' — a transient state of pulmonary hyper-inflation found immediately before total bronchial obstruction leads to collapse.
4 Signs of pneumonic infection distal to the tumour. Because of the bronchial obstruction breath sounds are usually reduced and bronchial breath sounds are rarely, if ever, heard in association with pneumonia distal to carcinoma.

N.B. Bronchial breath sounds are only heard over consolidation when the bronchi are fully patent.

Abnormal physical findings due to pleural involvement

1 Pleural effusion.
2 Pleural friction rub — sometimes in the absence of pleuritic pain.

Investigation of a patient with possible carcinoma of bronchus

Carcinoma of bronchus and its complications can produce symptoms which mimic all respiratory diseases and most disorders of other systems. The diagnosis must be considered in all adults, especially cigarette smokers, who present with the various features described above and summarized in Table 10.1. In such patients the investigations are aimed at:

1 Establishing a clinical diagnosis.
2 Determining the feasibility of 'curative' therapy. This involves:
   (i)   Establishing a pathological diagnosis.
   (ii) The exclusion or confirmation of metastatic disease.
   (iii) Evaluation of the risks of therapy.

It follows that the investigations undertaken will depend not only upon the presenting features, but also on such factors as the patient's age, general condition and physical signs both within and outwith the respiratory system.

Staging of bronchial carcinoma.   Staging is essentially a formalized way of assessing the operability of a tumour, and hence is not really applicable to small cell carcinomas which are usually inoperable at the

Table 10.1   Features requiring appropriate investigations to exclude carcinoma of the bronchus

Respiratory symptoms	X-ray abnormalities	Other features
Cough	Unilateral hilar prominence	Finger clubbing
Haemoptysis		Mediastinal problems
Breathlessness	Pulmonary collapse	Abnormalities
Wheeze	Peripheral shadow	suggesting distant
Hoarseness	Cavitated lesion	metastases (e.g. bone
Poorly resolving pneumonia	Pleural effusion	pain, focal fits)
Recurrent pneumonia		Non-specific symptoms of disease (e.g. weight loss)

time of presentation. Non-small cell carcinomas can be staged by a complicated system which uses T (tumour), N (nodes) and M (metastases) categories. (T N M classification) In brief, stage I and II tumours are small and stage III carcinomas are large and extend into neighbouring structures or into proximal main bronchi. Evidence of lymphatic and distant metastatic spread is also staged using the N and M categories. Tumours staged as T1 (or 2), N0, M0 carry the best prognosis, particularly if they are of squamous cell type, provided the patient is fit for thoracotomy.

Radiological examination

Radiology is of paramount importance in the diagnosis and the planning of treatment (Figs. 10.2 & 10.3).

STRAIGHT AND LATERAL CHEST X-RAYS

Normal chest X-ray does not exclude a bronchial tumour. Carcinomas in the larger bronchi, which may present with haemoptysis, may not be associated with any abnormality, because the mediastinal structures do not allow radiographic visualization of these centrally situated tumours.

ABNORMAL HILAR SHADOW

Enlargement of one hilum is probably the commonest X-ray abnormality. It may be due to the primary tumour or glandular metastases from a peripheral lesion. Early enlargement is difficult to detect and tomography (p. 22) may be of considerable value. A lateral film is always necessary since apparent hilar enlargement can arise from superimposition of a peripheral tumour in the apical segment of the lower lobe.

COLLAPSE OF SEGMENT, LOBE OR LUNG

Radiological evidence of segmental, lobar or total lung collapse is a frequent finding. However, it must be emphasized that a small tumour may be large enough to cause bronchial obstruction and hence be responsible for a major radiographic abnormality. The term collapse/consolidation is often used to describe the radiographic features produced by bronchial obstruction but true consolidation (opacification of the lung without evidence of collapse) is rare.

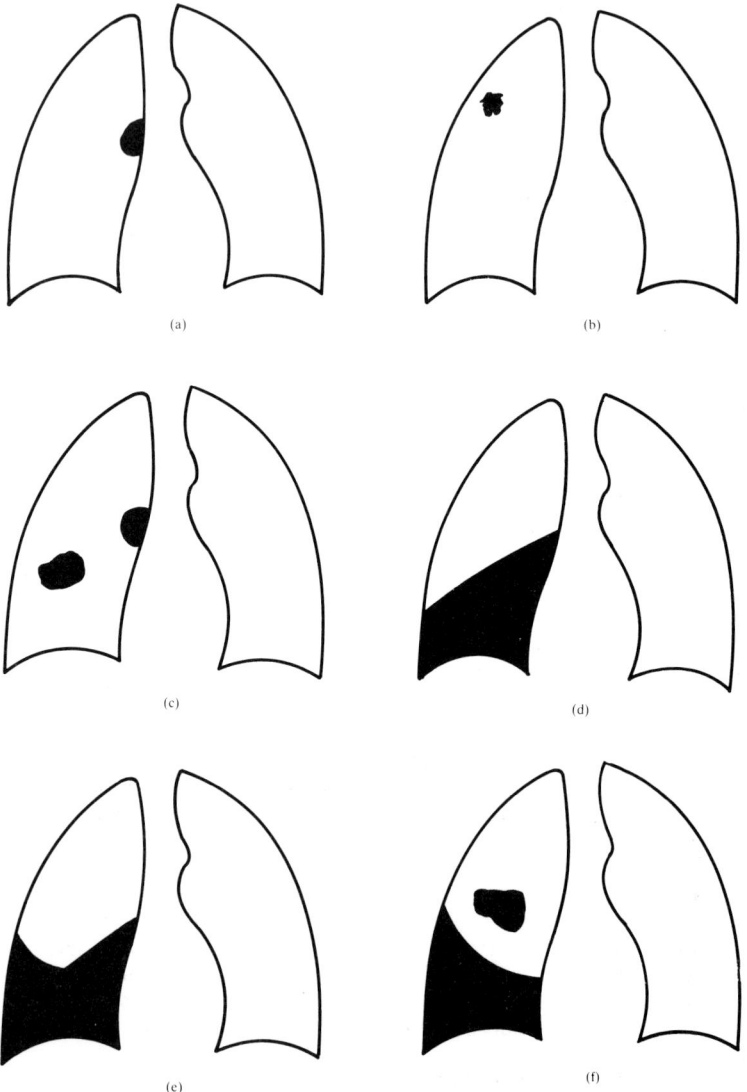

Fig. 10.2 Diagrammatic representation of X-ray presentations of bronchial carcinoma: (a) hilar enlargement, (b) peripheral pulmonary shadow, (c) peripheral pulmonary shadow and hilar enlargement. (d) pulmonary collapse, (e) pulmonary collapse and pleural effusion, (f) peripheral pulmonary shadow and pleural effusion.

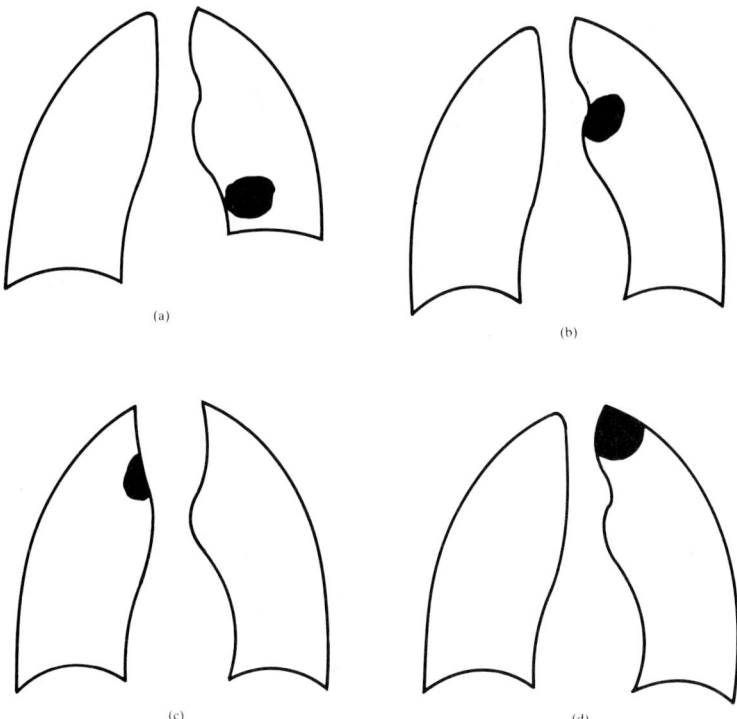

Fig. 10.3 Diagrammatic representation of X-ray presentations of bronchial carcinoma. (a) Pulmonary shadow adjacent to mediastinal structures and an elevated hemidiaphragm indicating phrenic nerve involvement. (b) Pulmonary shadow in relation to the aortic knuckle. This is the usual site of the tumour when there is hoarseness and bovine cough due to left recurrent laryngeal involvement. (c) Pulmonary shadow (and often evidence of hilar glandular enlargement) together with superior mediastinal widening. Patients with these X-ray abnormalities often have superior vena caval obstruction. (d) Pulmonary shadow in the apex of the lung (often with evidence of rib destruction). Tumours in this site may give rise to the clinical features of a 'Pancoast tumour'.

OBSTRUCTIVE EMPHYSEMA

Obstructive emphysema may be observed in cases where bronchial occlusion is not quite complete and is best confirmed by screening. During fluoroscopic examination the affected lobe or lung is hypertranslucent and does not deflate on expiration, which causes displacement of the mediastinum to the opposite side.

PERIPHERAL X-RAY SHADOW

Peripheral X-ray shadow due to a carcinoma may be small or huge and can have a smooth or irregular margin. Cavitation within a primary tumour is not uncommon (particularly with squamous carcinomas) and may only be demonstrated by tomography (p. 22).

PLEURAL EFFUSIONS

Malignant effusions are usually large.

PERICARDIAL EFFUSION

This is not uncommon.

MEDIASTINAL WIDENING

Widening of the upper mediastinum is common and massive widening is a feature of superior vena caval obstruction.

MULTIPLE PULMONARY ABNORMALITIES

Multiple large and small opacities are seen when the tumour has metastasized to other parts of the lung (pulmonopulmonary metastases). Widespread streaky shadows radiating from the hila, and usually associated with evidence of lymphatic obstruction (Kerley's B lines or septal lines) in the lower zones, are seen in cases when tumour spreads from mediastinal glands to pulmonary lymphatics (lymphatic carcinomatosis).

BONE DESTRUCTION

Destruction of bony structures, usually the ribs, can be seen when a peripheral tumour has directly invaded the chest wall or when a metastatic deposit has involved the ribs.

SCREENING OF THE LUNGS, HEMIDIAPHRAGMS

X-ray screening is an essential preoperative investigation. Paradoxical movement of a hemidiaphragm reflecting phrenic nerve involvement can only be satisfactorily demonstrated by screening. When the patient

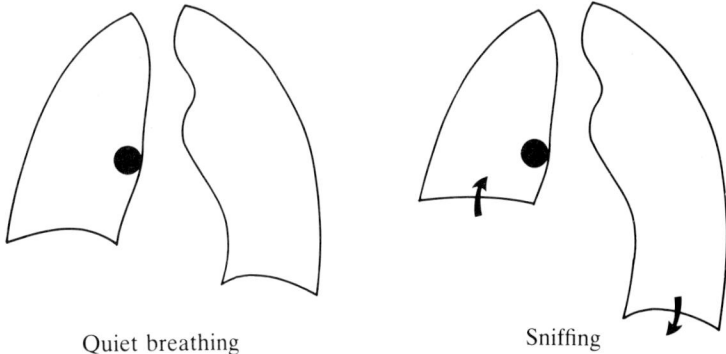

Quiet breathing   Sniffing

Fig. 10.4   Diagrammatic representation of fluoroscopic findings in patients with an elevated left hemidiaphragm due to phrenic nerve paralysis. Left hemidiaphragm is elevated but does not appear to move during quiet breathing. However, when the patient sniffs, the normal hemidiaphragm moves sharply down and the denervated side moves up (paradoxical movement).

sniffs the affected hemidiaphragm moves up sharply as the normal side goes down (Fig. 10.4). Screening is also very useful in the confirmation of obstructive emphysema, (*see* above).

BARIUM SWALLOW

Barium swallow is conveniently performed at the same time as screening. Separate views of the barium-filled oesophagus should be obtained in the straight, lateral and both oblique positions. However, a normal barium swallow does not exclude tumour invasion of the mediastinum. Tumour involvement, in particular of the subcarinal glands, may cause indentation of the oesophageal outline and thus indicate that surgical resection of all tumour tissue is not possible. Gross oesophageal compression is found in patients who present with dysphagia.

RADIOISOTOPE SCANNING

The place of radioisotope scanning of the lungs in the routine investigation of bronchial carcinoma is not yet established. Perfusion scans may be of some value in the differentiation between a primary bronchial carcinoma and a single metastatic deposit (much larger scan abnormalities are usually found in primary tumours) and perhaps in the detection of spread of tumour to the mediastinum. Liver, brain and bone scans are of value in the assessment of patients with small cell carcinoma and also in staging of patients with non-small cell tumours. However, examination of the liver by ultrasound is probably preferable to an isotope liver scan and CT scanning of the brain is far superior to an isotope scan.

COMPUTERIZED AXIAL TOMOGRAPHY (CT scanning)

CT scanning is of value in the staging of malignant disease of the thorax. Pulmonary metastatic deposits from a primary bronchial tumour not visible on conventional X-rays may be detected by CT and lymphatic spread to the mediastinum can also be investigated. However, this technique has not proved to be as useful as initially expected and is not readily available in many hospitals for the routine investigation of patients with bronchial carcinoma.

LIVER ULTRASONOGRAPHY

Ultrasonographic examination of the liver is a non-invasive, sensitive and quick way of detecting metastatic hepatic deposits. If necessary, biopsy of an abnormal area of echoeity can be performed under ultrasound control. Ultrasonographic examination of the liver has virtually replaced isotope liver scanning in the investigation of bronchial carcinoma.

BONE MARROW ASPIRATION AND TREPHINE BIOPSY

The examination of bone marrow and trephine bone marrow biopsies is an important pretreatment investigation of patients with small cell carcinoma who are being considered for aggressive chemotherapy or surgery.

Investigations

BRONCHOSCOPY

In most patients bronchoscopy is a vital investigation in order to establish the histological diagnosis and to determine whether the tumour is operable. Even small tumours close to the tracheal bifurcation are inoperable, since resection cannot be successfully performed unless there is 2 cm or more of normal bronchus on the left side to allow complete removal of tumour and suture of the bronchial stump. Resection of right main bronchus tumour is anatomically less difficult. Widening of the main carina by subcarinal glands indicates quite massive tumour spread to the mediastinum, and paralysis of the left vocal cord (confirmation only possible during bronchoscopy under local anaesthesia) is also evidence of inoperability.

A rigid or fibreoptic instrument can be used. The fibrescope gives improved access to the upper lobar and all segmental bronchi so that forceps, bronchial brush or lavage material can be obtained more easily from peripheral lesions. However, biopsies obtained with the fibreoptic instrument are very much smaller than those which can be taken via the rigid bronchoscope which also allows much more efficient suction (p. 30).

SPUTUM CYTOLOGY

The confident recognition of malignant cells in sputum is difficult and the value of this investigation is directly dependent upon the skills of the cytologist. An able cytologist can identify malignant cells in the sputum of the majority of patients with bronchial carcinoma, providing good sputum specimens are submitted for examination. Fresh sputum is ideal and some cytologists will refuse to examine sputum which has been expectorated more than a few hours before it reaches the laboratory. However, 24-hour sputum collections are preferred by others. At bronchoscopy, trap specimens of sputum, together with bronchial brushings and washings, should be taken from the abnormal lobe or segment and quickly submitted for cytological examination.

MEDIASTINOSCOPY (Fig. 10.5)

This relatively simple surgical procedure is valuable in the preoperative assessment of bronchial carcinoma as well as in the diagnosis of mediastinal abnormalities. The group of lymph glands around the trachea and main bronchi is accessible to mediastinoscopic examination and biopsy. Routine mediastinoscopy prior to thoracotomy decreases the number of operations at which the tumour is found to be inoperable by 10–20%. Mediastinoscopy carries a considerable risk of haemorrhage in patients with superior vena caval obstruction.

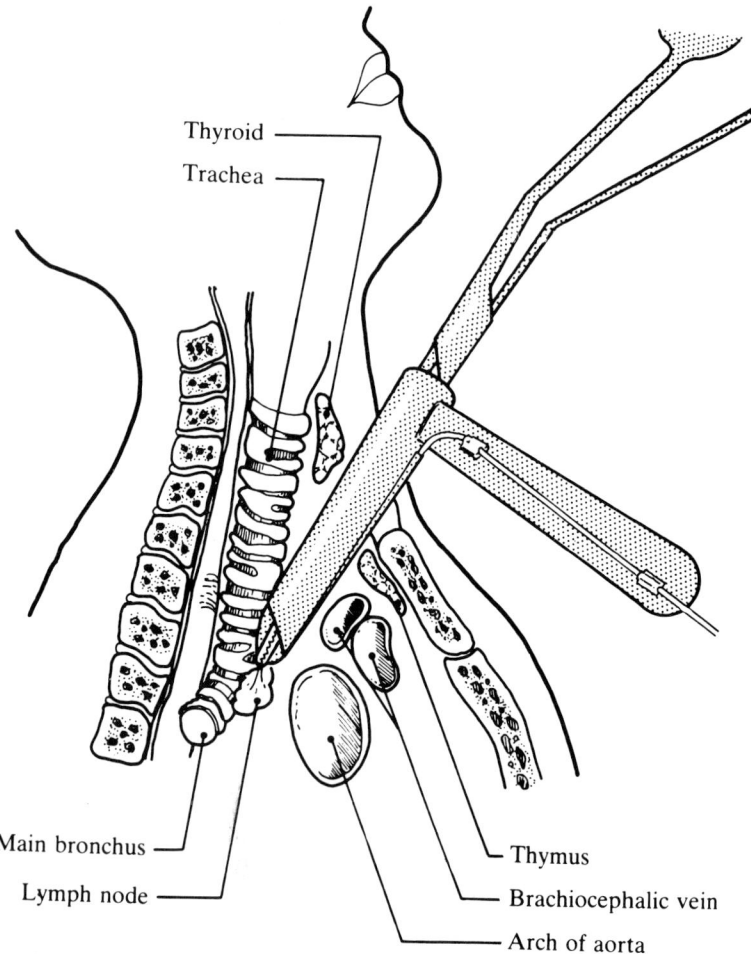

Thyroid

Trachea

Main bronchus

Lymph node

Thymus

Brachiocephalic vein

Arch of aorta

Fig. 10.5 Mediastinoscopy. Diagram of mediastinoscope in position anterior to the trachea allowing biopsy of a lymph node in the region of the main carina.

NECK GLAND BIOPSY

Tumour involvement of the scalene or other cervical nodes is absolute evidence of inoperability and aspiration or biopsy at an early stage is an essential part of investigation. Fine-needle aspiration of an enlarged node is a very simple procedure which, if positive, confirms the diagnosis and may prevent the need for more invasive investigations.

Differential diagnosis

The differential diagnoses are protean and depend upon the mode of presentation. The respiratory diseases most frequently simulated by carcinoma are:

1 Pneumonia and lung abscess.
2 Pulmonary tuberculosis.
3 Pulmonary infarction.
4 Bronchiectasis.
5 Metastatic pulmonary disease.
6 All the causes of diffuse pulmonary fibrosis (p. 212) have to be considered in the differential diagnosis of lymphatic carcinomatosis.

Treatment

Treatment can be either curative or palliative. Curative treatment is almost exclusively achieved by surgical resection, though radiotherapy is also effective in selected cases. Unfortunately, the majority of patients present with evidence of tumour spread and can only be offered palliative therapy. Radiotherapy, and in some cases chemotherapy, can usefully relieve distressing symptoms. Chemotherapy alone has not been successful in achieving cure but worthwhile increased survival times are now being reported in patients with small cell tumours.

Surgery

Resection of localized tumours gives the best results in terms of cure. However, few patients are suitable for surgery, and even in 'operable' patients the results are poor in undifferentiated and poorly differentiated tumours. In contrast, the five-year survival rate after resection of squamous carcinoma can be as high as 50%.

ROUTINE INVESTIGATIONS PRIOR TO THORACOTOMY

Assessment of ventilatory function

Many patients have poor ventilatory function because of associated chronic bronchitis and are unsuitable for surgical treatment because of high operative risks and the inevitable worsening of pulmonary function produced by the unavoidable removal of functioning lung tissue. In crude terms an FEV_1 of below one litre is a contraindication to thoracotomy and an FEV_1 of less than 1·2 litres, or a 12-minute walking distance of less than 1 km, are contraindications to pneumonectomy. It is rarely necessary to use more sophisticated tests of pulmonary function if the VFTs are assessed in conjunction with a careful clinical appraisal of dyspnoea.

Barium swallow and screening of hemidiaphragms

See p. 144.

Bronchoscopy

See p. 30.

Other investigations in selected patients

1   Neck gland biopsy (p. 148).
2   Mediastinoscopy (p. 148).
3   Liver scan and/or ultrasonic examination (p. 146).
4   Lung scan (p. 145).
5   Thoracoscopy (p. 32).

CONTRAINDICATIONS TO SURGICAL TREATMENT

1   Evidence of metastases (pleural, mediastinal or more widespread).
2   Poor respiratory function.
3   Other serious diseases (particularly heart disease).
4   Advanced age.
5   Small cell carcinoma (unless there is no evidence of extrapulmonary spread).

Radiotherapy (radical, curative)

Radiotherapy is less effective than surgey in squamous carcinoma and adenocarcinoma. Treatment results of undifferentiated tumours (e.g. small cell) are poor and at present treatment with chemotherapy is the treatment of choice if the tumour is inoperable. Combination of chemotherapy and radiotherapy appears to be no better than chemotherapy alone. Treatment with fast neutrons has not yet proved to be superior to conventional radiotherapy. Radiotherapy causes pulmonary damage and is not without risk in patients with poor pulmonary function.

Palliative radiotherapy

Palliative radiotherapy is of great value in improving quality of life, particularly in patients with localized bone pain, SVC obstruction, stridor and dysphagia.

Chemotherapy

Cure has not yet been reported, but much research is being undertaken in this field. It is hoped that treatment with combinations of cytotoxic drugs, perhaps together with immunotherapy, will be found to be more effective in the future. Several regimens are now being assessed.

Chemotherapy regimens

The combination of vindesine and etoposide (vindesine 3 mg/m^2 [maximum 5 mg] by bolus i.v. on day 1 and etoposide 120 mg/m^2 by i.v. infusion on days 2 and 3; six pulses of this treatment at three-week intervals) has minimal toxicity except for alopecia, and is almost as effective, as judged by remission rates and survival times, as much more toxic multiagent therapy with drugs such as cyclophosphamide, methotrexate and CCNU.

The discovery that mesna, a sulphydryl-containing compound, significantly reduces urotoxic effects (e.g. haemorrhagic cystitis) of the oxazaphosphorine alkylating agents such as cyclophosphamide and ifosfamide has allowed these alkylating agents to be given in higher doses.

Palliative chemotherapy

Like radiotherapy, chemotherapy can improve quality of life and is particularly useful in patients with widespread symptomatic disease, especially when caused by small cell carcinoma, which is too extensive for palliative radiotherapy.

If a malignant lesion is causing almost total obstruction of the trachea, i.v. ifosfamide 3–5 g/m^2 (maximum 10 g) with concurrent mesna (40% of dose of ifosfamide repeated after 3, 6 and 9 hours) together with oral prednisolone (20–40 mg daily) can be given before radiotherapy. Radiotherapy can induce initial tumour swelling which may be fatal in patients with almost total tracheal obstruction. Tumour swelling does not occur, or is not as great, after treatment with cytotoxic drugs and may be suppressed by corticosteroids.

Chemotherapeutic agents are used in the treatment of superior vena caval obstruction, dysphagia, etc., in small cell carcinoma, or when there is a contraindication to radiotherapy.

Chemotherapy can be expected to have an appreciable effect in small cell carcinoma and in some patients with undifferentiated large cell carcinoma, but the presently available drugs given alone or in combination have little or no effect on squamous and adenocarcinomas.

Laser treatment

Laser treatment via a fibreoptic bronchoscope is essentially palliative and is suitable for only a few patients with symptoms caused by a predominantly endobronchial tumour. The aim of treatment is to destroy tumour tissue occluding major airways and the best results are achieved in main bronchus tumours.

Prognosis

The overall prognosis in bronchial carcinoma is very poor (Table 10.2). Less than 10% of patients survive five years after prognosis. The best prognosis is with well-differentiated squamous tumours which have not metastasized and are amenable to surgical treatment. Resectable adenocarcinomas also have a relatively good prognosis, but with undifferentiated tumours the outlook is extremely poor since the various forms of treatment available are uniformly unsatisfactory, and very few patients survive for more than two years.

BRONCHIAL ADENOMA

General considerations including incidence

Bronchial adenomas are derived from the duct epithelium of bronchial mucous glands. They are often regarded as benign but most have low malignant propensities. These tumours are rare, being 50–100 times less common than bronchial carcinoma.

There are two main pathological types:

1 Carcinoid.
2 Cylindromatous.

The majority are carcinoid tumours. There is no relationship between bronchial adenoma and cigarette smoking.

Table 10.2 Summary of treatment related to tumour cell type.

	Squamous	Adenocarcinoma	Small cell	Large cell
Surgery	Best chance of cure.	Offers only chance of cure.	Rarely operable. Few cures reported.	Only rarely results in cure.
Radiotherapy	Radiosensitive. 'Curative' treatment worthwhile in patients not suitable for surgery. Palliative treatment helpful (bone pain, SVC obstruction, etc.).	Relatively insensitive to radiotherapy. 'Curative' treatment sometimes tried. Attempts to palliate always worthwhile.	Very radiosensitive. 'Curative' treatment rarely worthwhile because disease rarely localized. Palliative treatment useful. Radiotherapy used in combination with drugs.	Usually very radiosensitive but few patients cured. Palliative treatment useful.
Chemotherapy	Almost totally unresponsive.	Almost completely unresponsive.	Majority respond dramatically initially but rapidly relapse. Survival increased by chemotherapy.	Some response but not enough to justify widespread use of chemotherapy.

Fundamental points of diagnosis and complications

There are no specific features of bronchial adenoma. The presenting symptoms are the same as those produced by local effects of bronchial carcinoma — except that they tend to occur in a younger age group. Cough, recurrent haemoptysis and repeated pneumonias in the same site are the commonest presentations. However, since adenomas, particularly carcinoid types, tend to occur in larger bronchi, breathlessness associated with stridor may be the presentation. Physical signs, when present, relate to bronchial obstruction. Carcinoid syndrome and symptoms of metastatic spread are very rare.

Investigations

X-rays may be normal or show signs of partial (obstructive emphysema) or total bronchial occlusion (collapse). Peripheral lung shadows are less common. The majority of adenomas are visible at bronchoscopy since they have a predilection for larger bronchi. They may be mulberry-shaped and bleed freely when manipulated at bronchoscopy. Biopsy is usually more difficult than with carcinomas because the tumour mass is of firmer consistency and when pedunculated may be relatively mobile in the bronchus and difficult to grasp with biopsy forceps. Sputum cytology is of little or no value.

Differential diagnosis

In middle-aged and elderly patients a diagnosis of carcinoma is almost invariably made, and bronchoscopy with biopsy is necessary to establish the diagnosis of adenoma. In younger age groups the differential diagnosis is usually that of any disease which can cause repeated haemoptysis and pulmonary infection — notably bronchiectasis.

Treatment

Treatment whenever feasible is by surgical resection of tumour. In patients unfit for thoracotomy removal of the tumour tissue at bronchoscopy or laser treatment may restore a bronchial lumen, but this procedure rarely results in cure and has, therefore, to be repeated. Radiotherapy is of little use but should be tried in patients with unresectable tumours (e.g. adenoma causing tracheal obstruction) especially of cylindromatous type.

Prognosis

Prognosis is generally good and cure is usual in patients in whom the tumour can be resected. Carcinoid adenomas have a better prognosis than cylindromatous tumours.

BRONCHIOLOALVEOLAR CELL CARCINOMA (ALVEOLAR CARCINOMA)

General considerations including incidence

Bronchioloalveolar cell carcinoma is the least common primary carcinoma of the respiratory tract. It arises from the alveolar epithelium, probably type II alveolar cells, tends to grow along rather than invade pulmonary tissues, and may be multicentric in origin. It is somewhat less frequent than bronchial adenoma and approximately 100 times less common than bronchial carcinoma. The age incidence is the same as that of bronchial carcinoma. Some pathologists believe bronchioloalveolar cell carcinoma to be a form of adenocarcinoma.

Fundamental points of diagnosis

Many patients have no symptoms and the lesion is detected by routine radiography. When symptoms are present they are similar to those produced by bronchial carcinoma. The production of copious amounts of watery sputum has often been stressed as a diagnostic feature of this disease, but this only occurs in a small proportion of cases and then usually when the disease is at an advanced stage.

Complications

Complications of bronchioloalveolar cell carcinoma are predominantly intrathoracic, since spread within the lungs is more common than distant metastatic dissemination. Progressive breathlessness and death from respiratory failure is relatively common.

Clinical findings

Symptoms and signs

Symptoms occur relatively late in the course of the disease. All the common symptoms of bronchial carcinoma can be produced by bronchioloalveolar cell carcinoma but productive cough and breathlessness are more frequent than haemoptysis.

Physical findings in the chest are usually absent unless the disease is far advanced or has spread to the pleura. Finger clubbing occurs in some cases but not all.

Radiological examination

There are no characteristic radiological features, but there is a tendency for the disease to be common in the upper lobes. The disease can appear as a solitary pulmonary shadow, multiple lung shadows (unilateral or bilateral) or extensive lung shadowing with or without cavitation. In cases of extensive pulmonary infiltration an 'air bronchogram' may be visible. Pleural effusion occurs but not as frequently as with bronchial carcinoma.

Investigations

Examination of sputum for malignant cells is a valuable investigation.

Bronchoscopy is relatively unhelpful but must be performed in order to exclude bronchial carcinoma. Transbronchial biopsy (using a fibreoptic bronchoscope) or percutaneous lung biopsy may be the only way of establishing a diagnosis other than by surgical resection of the lesion.

Differential diagnosis

Diagnosis is usually difficult. The solitary pulmonary nodule often looks like bronchial carcinoma, but more extensive disease can be mistaken for tuberculosis or suppurative pneumonia.

Treatment

Surgical resection of isolated pulmonary lesions offers the only chance of cure. Bronchioloalveolar cell carcinoma is not favourably influenced by radiotherapy or chemotherapy.

Prognosis

The overall prognosis is better than that of bronchial carcinoma, because surgical resection gives somewhat better results and even when no treatment is possible the course of the disease may be slow, even though relentless.

OTHER TUMOURS

Tumours other than bronchial carcinoma, adenoma and bronchioloalveolar cell carcinoma are very uncommon.

Malignant reticuloses

These may occasionally arise in the bronchial lymph glands without evidence of disease elsewhere in the body. More commonly the mediastinal nodes, lungs and pleura are involved together with other organs in generalized disease. Occasionally patients with lymphoma may present with disease confined to the lung.

Pulmonary hamartoma

This simple tumour usually presents as a symptomless rounded peripheral pulmonary lesion on routine X-ray, and the diagnosis is made after surgical removal. The prognosis is excellent.

Others

Simple and malignant tumours of all the tissue elements of the bronchopulmonary system, such as chondroma, fibroma, lipoma, plasmacytoma and sarcoma do occur but are very rare indeed.

SECONDARY TUMOURS OF THE LUNG

Blood-borne pulmonary metastatic deposits are common and can arise from malignant tumours anywhere in the body. The most common primary sites are breast, kidney, ovary, testes and gut. Respiratory symptoms are uncommon unless lung tissue is extensively replaced by tumour or pleural effusion has developed. Occasionally metastatic lesions in the bronchi can produce the clinical and radiographic features usually associated with primary bronchial carcinoma.

MANAGEMENT OF SOLITARY PERIPHERAL X-RAY SHADOW

The most likely causes are:

1 Carcinoma — almost always primary since single metastatic deposits are uncommon.
2 Tuberculous lesion (active or quiescent).
3 Simple inflammatory lesion.
4 Rare causes e.g. simple tumour, rheumatoid nodule.

Previous chest X-rays

The examination of previous chest X-rays when available is of great value. If the lesion is present on a film taken years previously it can be assumed to be benign and no further investigations may be necessary, except perhaps for X-ray follow-up.

Antibiotic therapy

When no previous X-ray is available or if it is normal it is often sound practice to give an antibiotic (e.g. ampicillin) *while* other investigations are performed. Repeat X-ray at a week or 10 days will show reduction in size or clearing if it is a simple inflammatory lesion.

Routine investigations

1 Tuberculin test.
2 Examination of sputum for tubercle bacilli.
3 Examination of sputum for malignant cells.

Other investigations

Tomography (p. 22) may be helpful by demonstrating calcification or cavitation within the lesion and by defining its edge with greater clarity.

Barium swallow and screening of the hemidiaphragms should be performed in an attempt to detect evidence of mediastinal involvement by a malignant lesion.

Computerized axial tomography (CT).   It is claimed that measurement of the tissue attenuation of the solitary pulmonary nodule can indicate the likelihood of malignancy, higher 'attenuation units' being found in benign lesions compared with malignant tumours. CT can also identify second or multiple nodular lesions in metastatic disease which may not be visible on radiographs or be picked up by conventional tomography.

Histological diagnosis

In the majority of cases the diagnosis will remain uncertain in spite of the investigations outlined above and a definitive diagnosis can only be achieved by biopsy or resection of the abnormality.

Biopsy

1 *Fibreoptic bronchoscopy and transbronchial biopsy* using fluoroscopic control.
2 *Percutaneous biopsy* using fluoroscopic control.

Surgical resection

Providing there are no contraindications, such as advanced age or poor lung function, surgical resection of the lesion is indicated if a diagnosis has not been established or in selected patients in whom a diagnosis of primary carcinoma has been made. Single metastatic pulmonary tumours should be resected if possible in patients in whom the primary lesion was apparently successfully treated surgically and, of course, if there is no evidence of recurrence of disease elsewhere.

Other measures

Chemotherapy may be the treatment of choice if a diagnosis of anaplastic carcinoma has been made or if the patient is unfit for operation. Radiotherapy can be used in patients in whom there is a contraindication to surgery.

Antituberculosis therapy. In some patients unfit for thoracotomy it may be prudent to give antituberculosis treatment (usually isoniazid and rifampicin). Decrease in size of the lesion during treatment suggests tuberculosis, whereas increase in size excludes this diagnosis.

SUMMARY — SPECIAL POINTS OF EMPHASIS

• Bronchial carcinoma is common.

- Over 90% of patients die within five years of diagnosis.

- It is often symptomless until a late stage.

- Cough and scanty haemoptysis are the most common symptoms.

- Breathlessness is usually due to bronchial obstruction and/or pleural effusion.

- Finger clubbing is more often due to bronchial carcinoma than any other condition.

- Careful examination of the neck is essential, since spread to scalene nodes indicates widespread tumour involvement of mediastinum.

- A normal chest X-ray does not exclude bronchial carcinoma.

- A large chest X-ray abnormality due to collapse of lung distal to a tumour can be caused by a small operable tumour.

- Physical signs in the chest are commonly absent when the tumour has not caused bronchial obstruction or pleural effusion.

- Bronchial breath sounds are rarely heard in patients with carcinoma of bronchus.

- Bronchoscopy is an essential investigation in most patients.

- Tuberculosis, pneumonia and simple lung abscess can be simulated by bronchial carcinoma.

- Treatment of bronchial carcinoma, except for surgical resection of localized squamous tumours, is unsatisfactory.

- Palliative treatment of symptoms such as bone pain, superior vena caval obstruction, etc. can improve quality of life enormously.

- The treatment of choice for inoperable small cell carcinoma is chemotherapy.

Further reading

Bates M. (1984) *Bronchial Carcinoma. An Integrated Approach to Diagnosis and Management*. Berlin: Springer–Verlag.
Cameron E. (1983) Surgical aspects of lung cancer. *Hospital Update* **9**, 429–41.
Choi N.C. & Grillo H.C. (Eds.) (1983) *Thoracic Oncology*. New York: Raven Press.

Dunlop D. & Harvey J. (1982) The solitary pulmonary nodule. *Brit. J. Hosp. Med.* 138–46.

Howard G.C.W. & Bleehan N.M. (1983) Pancoast's syndrome. *Brit. J. Hosp. Med.* **29**, 496–503.

Mountain C.F. (1977) Assessment of the role of surgery for control of lung cancer. *Ann. thorac. Surg.* **24**, 365–73.

Smyth J.F. (1984) *The Management of Lung Cancer.* London: Edward Arnold.

Strauss M.J. (1977) *Lung Cancer: Clinical Diagnosis and Treatment.* New York: Grune & Stratton.

Chapter 11
Diseases of the pleura

General considerations

Primary diseases of the pleura are uncommon but pleural involvement frequently complicates pulmonary diseases. Pleural diseases, whether primary or secondary, produce similar symptoms and physical signs. It is convenient to discuss diseases of the pleura (other than pneumothorax, *see* p. 176) under the headings of: (a) pleurisy; (b) pleural effusion and empyema; (c) pleural tumours, fibrosis and calcification. However, this should not be regarded as a classification of pleural diseases.

PLEURISY

Pleurisy is not a diagnosis but is simply the term used to describe any pathological process which involves the pleura and gives rise to pleuritic pain or clinical evidence of pleural friction. The diseases which cause pleurisy are capable of producing pleural effusion. 'Dry pleurisy' is frequently used to describe pleurisy without pleural effusion, but this is not a satisfactory term since almost all causes of pleural effusion may produce 'dry pleurisy' before the development of effusion.

The commonest causes of pleurisy are pulmonary infections (pneumonia), pulmonary infarction, tuberculosis and bronchial carcinoma. Primary malignant disease of the pleura (mesothelioma) is uncommon compared with bronchial carcinoma, but produces pleurisy at an early stage. Metastatic pulmonary malignant disease is frequently associated with pleural involvement. Connective tissue disorders such as rheumatoid disease and systemic lupus erythematosus are rare causes of pleurisy. Very occasionally the often diagnosed but rarely confirmed epidemic myalgia (Bornholm disease) is accompanied by true pleurisy. Chest wall trauma may involve the pleura and evidence of pleurisy may very rarely be found in patients with uraemia. Eosinophilic pleurisy is extremely rare as is right-sided pleurisy as a manifestation of gonococcal disease (Fitz-Hugh and Curtis syndrome).

Fundamental points of diagnosis

Pleurisy can be diagnosed in any patient who has pleuritic pain or a pleural friction rub. Pleural pain is characteristically knife-like and made worse by deep breathing and coughing. It is rarely central and is easily distinguished from other types of chest pain, except musculo-skeletal chest wall disorders, especially fractured ribs. Pleural friction may not be audible in all patients with pleuritic pain and conversely pleural pain may be absent in patients found to have pleural friction.

Complications

The common local complication of pleurisy is the development of pleural effusion. Empyema and pneumothorax are rare and other complications are dependent upon the nature of the underlying disease causing the pleurisy.

Clinical findings

Symptoms and signs

There may be features of the underlying disease (e.g. pneumonia, pulmonary infarction) but the dominant symptom is pleuritic pain, which can occasionally be bilateral. Chest expansion at the site of pain is restricted and breath sounds are diminished. There may be signs of underlying pulmonary pathology such as crepitations and bronchial breathing, but the diagnostic feature is the pleural friction rub. Pain often restricts chest movement so much that a rub cannot be heard until pain has been eased by a potent analgesic. Pleural rubs are characteristically increased by deep breathing. When pleuropericardial friction is present the rub is synchronous with cardiac systole and is also augmented by breathing. Patients with pleuritic pain are often breathless because they breathe quickly and shallowly to avoid aggravating their pain.

Investigations

All investigations are performed in order to discover the underlying cause of pleurisy. Chest X-ray is the most important. If normal a diagnosis of 'dry pleurisy' may be made, but a normal X-ray does not exclude an associated pulmonary disease.

Differential diagnosis

The differential diagnosis of pleuritic pain in a patient without an obvious underlying pulmonary abnormality includes fractured rib, intercostal myalgia, costochondritis, herpes zoster and other causes of pain of intercostal nerve distribution such as compression fracture of a mid or upper thoracic vertebral body. Occasionally acute upper abdominal disease such as cholecystitis, pancreatitis or subphrenic infection may simulate pleuritic pain.

Malignant involvement of the chest wall may be present as well as malignant pleurisy. The pain of chest wall invasion is usually a constant dull ache, but may be made worse by breathing and coughing.

Treatment

Specific treatment is of the cause of pleurisy, but in all patients it is essential to give adequate analgesic therapy to relieve pleuritic pain. Usually pethidine (100 mg i.m.) or morphine (10 mg i.m.) is necessary. Adequate relief of pain is essential to allow patients to co-operate with the physiotherapist.

Prognosis

The prognosis in individual cases depends upon the cause (*see* Pleural effusion).

PLEURAL EFFUSION

Pleural effusion can be defined as the exudation or transudation of fluid into the pleural space in clinically (or radiographically) recognizable amounts. Like pleurisy, pleural effusion is a 'sign' of disease and not a diagnosis. Traditionally pleural effusion is often reserved for the description of serous effusions (exudates) and not applied to a low protein-containing collection of pleural fluid (transudate), as found in cardiac failure, or the purulent effusion (empyema). However, the clinical differentiation of these different types of pleural accumulations of fluid is often impossible before a sample of pleural liquid has been obtained by aspiration.

Virtually all causes of pleurisy may lead to the development of a pleural effusion (exudate). A pleural transudate or hydrothorax may be found in cardiac failure, constrictive pericarditis and hypoproteinaemic states such as nephrotic syndrome and hepatic cirrhosis. Myxoedema can be complicated by hydrothorax and an even rarer cause is ovarian tumour, usually fibroma, also associated with ascites (Meigs' syndrome). Empyema most often is caused by extension of infection from the lung, but can also be a complication of a penetrating injury of the chest wall or thoracotomy. Occasionally an empyema may develop by spread of infection from below the diaphragm and can also result from the introduction of pathogenic organisms into any sterile effusion or hydrothorax during diagnostic procedures.

Chylothorax can develop as a result of injury or malignant involvement of the thoracic duct.

Haemothorax is usually the result of trauma, and is often accompanied by pneumothorax. Malignant effusions are frequently haemorrhagic, as may be effusions related to pulmonary infarction.

Fundamental points of diagnosis

The only symptom of pleural effusion is breathlessness. Small accumulations of pleural fluid may not be detectable clinically but are usually visible radiographically. When effusion has been confirmed radiographically pleural aspiration should be performed if the underlying cause is in doubt. Pleural effusion often complicates bacterial pneumonia when it is usually associated with increase or recurrence of pyrexia in spite of apparently effective antibiotic treatment.

Complications

By and large the complications of an effusion are the complications of the underlying pathological process. A large pleural effusion causes compression of the lung and impairment of pulmonary function which is usually evident clinically by breathlessness. A serous effusion accompanying pulmonary infection may become infected and form an empyema. Rarely an empyema may discharge itself spontaneously through the chest wall (empyema necessitasis), or into a bronchus, resulting in cough productive of large amounts of pus and the development of a bronchopleural fistula, which shows on the chest X-ray as a 'fluid level' in the pleural space (pyopneumothorax).

Clinical findings

Symptoms and signs

Symptoms of the underlying disease are usually present. When progressive exertional breathlessness is the only presenting feature the most likely cause is malignant disease. Pleuritic pain often precedes the development of an effusion, but the separation of the visceral and parietal pleural layers by fluid relieves the pain and abolishes pleural friction. Pleural pain may recur after aspiration or spontaneous resolution of pleural fluid.

The physical signs of pleural effusion are, in the main, readily elicited unless the effusion is small. Loculated effusions in fissures between lobes often do not produce abnormal signs, and loculations above the diaphragm or against the chest wall may be difficult to detect clinically. A large effusion in a pleural space free from adhesions causes decreased chest expansion and mediastinal displacement to the opposite side. The percussion note is stony dull and breath sounds absent or decreased. Vocal resonance and fremitus are also decreased. In a few cases bronchial breath sounds are audible over the upper level of dullness, even in the absence of underlying pulmonary consolidation.

Radiological examination

Loculated effusions can cause radiological abnormalities which may be difficult to interpret but usually a pleural effusion is obvious on the chest X-ray. Small effusions may cause obliteration of the costophrenic angle but effusions of any size produce a homogeneous density in the lower part of the hemithorax with a concave upper margin. The X-ray usually suggests more fluid in the lateral (axillary) part of the chest but this is simply an X-ray artefact (for explanation of shape of pleural effusion see Fig. 11.1). Very large effusions completely fill the hemithorax and cause uniform opacification of one side. Most large effusions cause mediastinal displacement to the opposite side which is readily seen on the X-ray (Fig. 11.2); absence of mediastinal displacement indicates underlying collapse. Effusions may be bilateral and the X-ray may show evidence of underlying pulmonary disease. The lateral view is useful in locating the site of loculated effusions.

Investigations

The most important investigations of pleural effusions are examination of pleural fluid obtained by aspiration, and pleural biopsy. Following aspiration the chest radiograph should be repeated, since removal of pleural fluid may allow visualization of pulmonary and pleural lesions previously obscured by the effusion. During aspiration and pleural biopsy air is sometimes inadvertently introduced into the pleural space, but rarely in sufficient amounts to require treatment. Air in the pleural

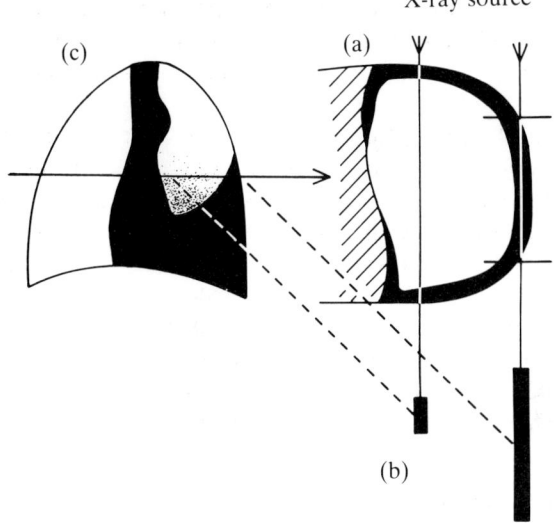

Fig. 11.1   A = Horizontal section of hemithorax at upper limit of effusion.
B = 'Columns' of fluid encountered by X-ray beams.
C = X-ray appearance of pleural effusion.

space can help to delineate pleural tumours otherwise not clearly visible
on X-ray. Air has to be deliberately introduced into the pleural space
prior to thoracoscopy (*see below*).

EXAMINATION OF PLEURAL FLUID

Naked eye inspection

Clear pleural fluid ranges in colour from light yellow to deep amber.
Cloudy fluid indicates a high cell content, usually polymorphs, or the
presence of cholesterol or fat droplets. Cholesterol crystals produce a
characteristic shimmering effect when the fluid is shaken and examined
in bright light. Fat droplets in a chylous effusion are responsible for the
opalescent or milky appearance of the fluid. Frankly purulent fluid
(empyema) is readily recognizable, as is a haemorrhagic effusion.

Microscopic examination

Cytological examination is of great diagnostic importance. Samples of
pleural fluid should be examined for blood cells (differential cell count)

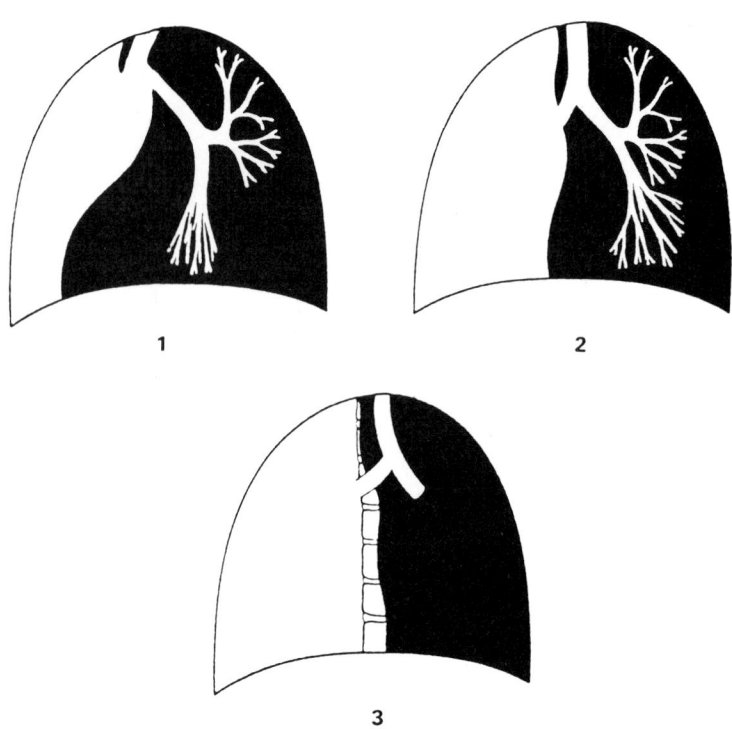

Fig. 11.2 Position of mediastinal structures in (1) massive pleural effusion, (2) consolidation of left lung, and (3) collapse of left lung (or pneumonectomy).

and also for malignant cells. All specimens of pleural fluid contain serosal cells derived from the pleura, and some blood cells. The identification of malignant cells is diagnostic, even though it may not be possible to determine the cell type of the tumour. A differential cell count is rarely diagnostic but often suggests a likely diagnosis: red cells predominate in effusions caused by malignant disease and pulmonary infarction; polymorphs suggest a bacterial cause (e.g. pneumonia); and lymphocytes are often, but not always, the predominant cell in tuberculous effusions. Eosinophils may be found in large numbers in any effusion which contains blood, but when there is a peripheral blood eosinophilia this may indicate a connective tissue disease or very rarely eosinophilic pleural effusion.

Biochemical investigations

Protein. A protein content of above 30 g/l indicates an exudate. Transudates have a low protein content of less than 30 g/l.

Glucose. A low glucose content is characteristically found in rheumatoid pleural effusions, but low levels compared with those present in the blood are also found in any effusions with high cellular activity (e.g. malignant and purulent effusions).

Cholesterol. Laboratory confirmation of the presence of cholesterol, which is often evident on naked eye inspection, simply indicates that the pleural effusion is chronic. Most chronic pleural effusions are caused by rheumatoid disease.

Fat. The presence of fat, which also is usually suggested by naked eye inspection, confirms chylothorax.

Amylase. Effusions complicating pancreatitis and sometimes carcinoma of the pancreas have very high amylase concentrations.

'Serological tests'

Effusions in patients with connective tissue disorders such as rheumatoid disease and systemic lupus erythematosus often contain rheumatoid factor and antinuclear factor. However, a positive finding must be interpreted with caution since a pleural effusion developing in a patient with rheumatoid disease is likely to contain rheumatoid factor, irrespective of the cause of the effusion.

Bacteriological examination

Rarely are pathogenic organisms visible on microscopy, but bacteriological culture of pleural fluid is indicated in all cases when an effusion complicates pneumonia. Appropriate anaerobic culture should be specifically requested whenever anaerobic infection is suspected, and likewise a specific request for mycological cultural methods should be made if a fungal cause is suspected. Whenever pleural fluid is submitted to the laboratory for examination for *Mycobacterium tuberculosis* as large a volume of fluid as possible should be sent.

PLEURAL BIOPSY

Biopsy of the parietal pleura can be easily performed at the same time as pleural aspiration using an Abrams pleural biopsy punch or modification of this aspiration/biopsy needle. Pleural biopsy is extremely valuable in the investigation of malignant and tuberculous effusions, since it provides much more chance of establishing a diagnosis than simple cytological and mycobacteriological examination of pleural fluid. If adequate specimens of pleura are obtained a diagnosis of malignant disease can be confirmed in up to 60% of patients, and in tuberculosis the chance of establishing a diagnosis is even higher. Pleural biopsy can also be useful in rarer conditions such as connective tissue disorders.

TECHNIQUE OF PLEURAL BIOPSY USING THE ABRAMS BIOPSY PUNCH

See Fig. 11.3. The position of the biopsy port A is indicated by the nipple on nut B. The biopsy port is closed by clockwise rotation of nut C and opened by anticlockwise rotation.

After local anaesthetic infiltration of the skin, chest wall and parietal pleura, the punch is introduced into the effusion through a small skin incision made with a scalpel. A large syringe (50 ml) and three-way tap is attached to the punch either before introduction into the chest or immediately afterwards. If the syringe is attached after insertion care must be taken to ensure the needle biopsy port is closed to avoid introduction of air into the chest.

Aspiration of pleural liquid for diagnostic purposes

The first stage is to remove pleural fluid for cytological, biochemical and bacteriological purposes. This should be done before biopsy to avoid contamination of the specimens with bleeding from the biopsy site(s).

Biopsy of parietal pleura

With the aid of the nipple on nut B the biopsy port is positioned (usually away from the mediastinum) and the needle and syringe are angled, using the chest wall as a fulcrum, and gradually withdrawn until the biopsy port is felt to engage parietal pleura. While the punch is kept in this position the biopsy port is closed by clockwise rotation of nut C.

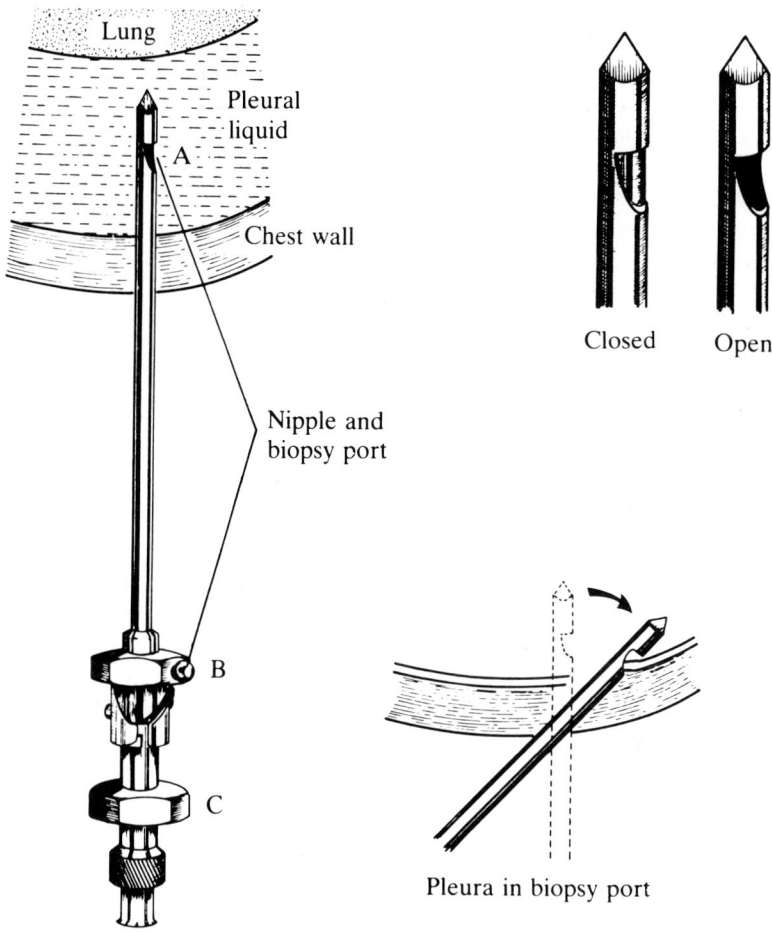

Closed   Open

Pleura in biopsy port

Fig. 11.3 Pleural biopsy using Abrams' pleural biopsy punch.

With the port closed the punch is then removed from the chest and the biopsied tissue is removed from the port. A number of biopsies can be obtained from different positions around the original entry site. Damage to the intercostal vessels can be avoided by taking biopsies below the horizontal.

Aspiration of pleural liquid for therapeutic purposes

Finally the biopsy punch is introduced into the pleural effusion again so that pleural liquid can be removed as necessary for therapeutic purposes.

    N.B. 1   The Abrams' biopsy punch should not be used to biopsy pleura when a pleural effusion is not present.

         2   Biopsy can be safely performed only when the port of the needle is in a pleural effusion as indicated by easy aspiration of pleural liquid.

Other procedures

Thoracoscopy may be necessary in some cases when a diagnosis has not been established by the methods already described. Very occasionally thoracotomy may have to be performed.

Differential diagnosis

Radiographically, loculated effusions can simulate pulmonary and pleural tumours and also elevation of a hemidiaphragm. Pleural fibrosis may occasionally produce clinical and radiological changes which are similar to those of pleural effusion.

Treatment

Treatment of a pleural effusion is removal of the fluid when indicated, usually by simple aspiration, combined with treatment of the underlying cause. Aspiration of a large effusion is sometimes necessary to relieve breathlessness but in the majority of cases aspiration (together with pleural biopsy) is performed for diagnostic reasons.

Malignant pleural effusion

In patients with small cell carcinoma systemic chemotherapy may effectively control a malignant effusion. However, in other malignancies there is rarely any specific treatment and pleurodesis (obliteration of the pleural space) is frequently indicated, as this may improve the quality of life by preventing the need for frequent pleural aspirations, which is the only effective way of controlling breathlessness. Pleurodesis can be performed in a number of ways, but probably the least upsetting to the patient is by the injection of 7–14 mg of inactivated *Corynebacterium parvum* into the pleural space immediately after aspiration of the pleural liquid. Repeat aspiration may be necessary within 48–72 hours of treatment, but often the fluid is loculated and aspiration is difficult. Intrapleural *C. parvum* often causes fever and occasionally there is quite marked systemic disturbance.

An alternative way of achieving pleurodesis which can also be used if *C. parvum* is not successful is performed in two stages using intrapleural mustine hydrochloride and intercostal intubation:

Stage 1. Aspiration of the bulk of the effusion followed by the injection of mustine hydrochloride 20 mg into the residual pleural fluid. The patient should then be encouraged to lie flat in prone and supine positions with the foot of the bed raised in order that the mustine can reach all parts of the pleural space. Since the intrapleural injection of mustine can cause pleural pain and nausea and vomiting parenteral pethidine (100 mg) and chlorpromazine (50–100 mg) should be given an hour or so before mustine is injected into the pleural space. Within 24 hours a chemical pleurisy is produced and the pleural surfaces are acutely inflamed. This is usually accompanied by rapid formation of pleural fluid.

Stage 2. The aim of stage 2 is to remove all pleural fluid so that the inflamed pleural surfaces are in contact and become adherent. Unless all fluid is removed complete pleurodesis cannot take place. For the removal of all fluid an intercostal tube is introduced through a low intercostal space, attached to an underwater seal drain and allowed to drain freely. The intercostal tube can usually be removed within 48 hours.

Empyema

Simple aspiration of an empyema is rarely completely successful unless the pus is thin. Repeated aspiration of as much pus as possible must be performed and accompanied by high-dose systemic antibiotic treatment. Even if the pus is thin it is probably best to use an intercostal tube to drain the pleural space effectively. Surgical treatment is indicated in all cases when pus is thick and is not readily drained by an intercostal tube. Drainage by rib resection will usually be chosen in the acute stage. Chronic empyema can be totally removed at thoracotomy.

Prognosis

The outcome depends upon the underlying cause. Malignant pleural effusions are associated with a very poor prognosis. The majority of effusions complicating pneumonia and pulmonary infarction respond rapidly to appropriate treatment and resolve completely. Empyema, although now rare, is still a serious disease which can prove fatal or produce considerable morbidity.

PLEURAL FIBROSIS, CALCIFICATION AND TUMOURS

Pleural fibrosis

Pleural fibrosis is usually the result of inadequately treated pleural effusion or empyema. Haemothorax may also lead to extensive pleural thickening. Extensive pleural fibrosis can be caused by drugs, e.g. methysergide and practolol. Pleural plaques associated with asbestos inhalation are described elsewhere (p. 205).

Extensive fibrosis of the pleura causes a restrictive defect, which if bilateral may be severely disabling. In some patients surgical removal of the thickened pleura (decortication) can be performed. There is no effective medical treatment. Drugs such as methysergide must, of course, be discontinued.

Pleural calcification

Calcification of the pleura is a very common radiographic finding, but is rarely sufficiently extensive to produce restriction of chest movement. The causes of pleural calcification are:

Tuberculosis
Non-tuberculous empyema
Haemothorax
Asbestos inhalation.

Pleural calcification has also been described in ankylosing spondylitis and in many patients the cause cannot be defined. Treatment is rarely necessary. If it is causing restriction of chest expansion decortication of the pleura should be considered.

Pleural tumours

Primary tumours of pleura are very rare compared with tumours of the bronchus. Malignant pleural tumours (malignant mesotheliomas) are much more common than benign lesions (fibromas or localized mesotheliomas).

Pleural fibroma (localized fibrous mesothelioma)

This rare tumour may be asymptomatic, but can cause chest pain, finger clubbing and hypertrophic pulmonary osteoarthropathy (p. 138). When asymptomatic it may be picked up on routine chest X-ray as a round or oval pleural opacity. When associated with symptoms the tumour, before thoracotomy, is often considered to be a malignant pleural tumour. Surgical removal results in dramatic relief of symptoms of hypertrophic pulmonary osteoarthropathy and slower resolution of finger clubbing.

Malignant mesothelioma

This tumour, derived from pleuromesothelial cells, is in the vast majority of cases caused by asbestos inhalation, usually some 35–40 years previously (p. 205). It spreads initially along the plane of the pleura, and in more than 80% of cases gives rise to a massive pleural effusion at an early stage, and, therefore, it usually presents initially with breathlessness. Spontaneous absorption of the fluid is quite common with time and the tumour then invades the chest wall and mediastinal structures. At this stage constant chest pain is the most common symptom. Pain down the arm from brachial plexus involvement may also be distressing. Hyperhydrosis followed by anhydrosis of one side of the chest, Horner's syndrome, and intercostal nerve root pain occur because of involvement of intercostal nerves and sympathetic ganglia. The tumour may be relatively slow-growing and the general condition of the patient may remain quite good for a considerable time in spite of intractable pain. Life expectancy from the time of diagnosis is, on average, a little over a year, but a minority survive 3–4 years.

Diagnosis is often suggested by X-ray manifestations of asbestos exposure (e.g. pleural plaques and pleural calcification) in a patient with a pleural effusion and/or chest pain. In such a case, particularly if there has been known asbestos exposure in the past, it may be wise to avoid trying to confirm the diagnosis by pleural aspiration, pleural biopsy, thoracoscopy or thoracotomy, since all these procedures usually result in seeding of the tumour to the chest wall. There is no treatment which favourably influences the progression of this unpleasant disease. The role of asbestos in its causation is accepted in law and it is now a prescribed disease. However medicolegal aspects should not be allowed to induce overzealous attempts to prove the diagnosis histologically, because of the risks of producing superficial chest wall tumour masses, which may ulcerate through the skin.

SUMMARY — SPECIAL POINTS OF EMPHASIS

• Primary diseases of the pleura are uncommon.

• The commonest causes of pleurisy are pulmonary infections, pulmonary infarction, tuberculosis and bronchial carcinoma.

• Pleuritic pain is usually severe and requires potent analgesic therapy such as pethidine or morphine.

• Pleural effusion is the exudation or transudation of fluid into the pleural space in clinically or radiographically recognizable amounts.

• Virtually all causes of pleurisy may lead to the development of pleural effusion.

• The clinical features of pleural effusion are breathlessness, decreased chest expansion, stony dull percussion note and absent air entry.

• In all cases of pleural effusion of unknown cause a pleural biopsy should be taken at the time of aspiration.

• The chest X-ray of a pleural effusion characteristically suggests that more fluid is present in the lateral part of the chest (i.e. 'goes up towards the axilla') — this is an X-ray artefact.

• The commonest causes of pleural calcification are tuberculosis, nontuberculous empyema, haemothorax and asbestos inhalation.

• Malignant pleural mesothelioma is, in the vast majority of cases, caused by asbestos inhalation.

Further reading

Dhillon D.P. & Spiro S.G. (1983) Malignant pleural effusions. *Brit. J. Hosp. Med.* **29**, 506–10.
Edge J.R. (1983) Mesothelioma. *Brit. J. Hosp. Med.* **29**, 521–36.
Howard G.C.W. & Bleehan N.M. (1983) *Pancoast's syndrome. Brit. J. Hosp. Med.* **29**, 496–503.
Lowell J.R. (1977) *Pleural Effusions: A Comprehensive Treatise.* Baltimore: University Park Press.

Chapter 12
Pneumothorax and mediastinal emphysema

INTRODUCTION

Pneumothorax is said to have occurred when the visceral and parietal pleural layers are separated by air. Air can reach the pleural space from the lung through a breach in the visceral pleura, or through the chest wall either from traumatic injury or during a surgical procedure.

Spontaneous pneumothorax is the term used to describe a pneumothorax which has developed in the absence of trauma or surgery. Air enters the pleural space through the visceral pleura and the elastic properties of the lung allow it to shrink to a size which is dependent upon the amount of air that has entered the pleural space and the presence or absence of adhesions between the visceral and parietal pleural layers. Thus, when a large volume of air enters a free pleural space the lung may recoil down to a small mass attached to the mediastinum at the pulmonary hilum; conversely, when only a small volume of air has escaped the two layers of pleura may be just separated. In the presence of pleural adhesions the lung is tagged to the parietal pleura at the sites of adhesions, but there may be large pneumothorax spaces where the pleura is free.

Open pneumothorax is a term used to indicate that the breach in the visceral pleura is still patent. The use of this term can lead to confusion, since in surgical parlance it is often taken to indicate a pneumothorax associated with a penetrating injury to the chest wall (traumatic pneumothorax).

Closed pneumothorax is a term used to indicate that the hole in the visceral pleura has become sealed off. Shallow pneumothoraces in the absence of pleural adhesions are 'closed'.

Tension pneumothorax. In a few cases the defect in the visceral pleura can form a flap valve type of mechanism and allow air to enter the pleural space on deep breathing and coughing, but not to re-enter the lung. During deep respiration and particularly coughing very high intra-pulmonary pressures are created. A pressure greater than atmospheric is built up within the pneumothorax and the mediastinum is displaced to the opposite side. Compression of the heart and great vessels may lead to circulatory collapse. It must be remembered that a tension pneumothorax may develop even though there are pleural adhesions present preventing total separation of the lung from the chest wall.

Traumatic pneumothorax can occur with penetrating injuries of the chest, rib fractures and ruptured bronchus. Accidental laceration of the visceral pleura may complicate procedures such as percutaneous lung biopsy, transbronchial lung biopsy, liver biopsy, pleural aspiration or biopsy, and also following cannulation of the great veins of the neck, e.g. CVP monitoring. All surgical operations involving thoracotomy are, of course, associated with pneumothorax.

Artificial pneumothorax.   The deliberate introduction of air into the pleural space was once a routine treatment for pulmonary tuberculosis. Rarely artificial pneumothorax may be of use diagnostically in the investigation of peripheral pleural or pulmonary lesions. Prior to thoracoscopy air must be introduced into the pleural space.

Haemopneumothorax, hydropneumothorax and pyopneumothorax indicate the presence of blood, clear pleural fluid or pus respectively as well as air in the pleural space.

Different types of pneumothorax are shown in Fig. 12.1.

SPONTANEOUS PNEUMOTHORAX

General considerations

Spontaneous pneumothorax can occur in patients who have apparently normal lungs. This type of pneumothorax is sometimes called 'pneumothorax simplex' and appears in young adults, usually males. The cause of the visceral pleural defect is assumed to be a bulla or bleb, which may be related to disease such as whooping cough in infancy.

Spontaneous pneumothorax complicates chronic obstructive airways disease, especially chronic bronchitis and emphysema, and many chronic diseases associated with pulmonary fibrosis, particularly when 'honeycomb lung' has been produced. Rupture of pulmonary cavities into the pleural space produces pneumothoraces in diseases such as suppurative pneumonia and tuberculosis. Very occasionally there may

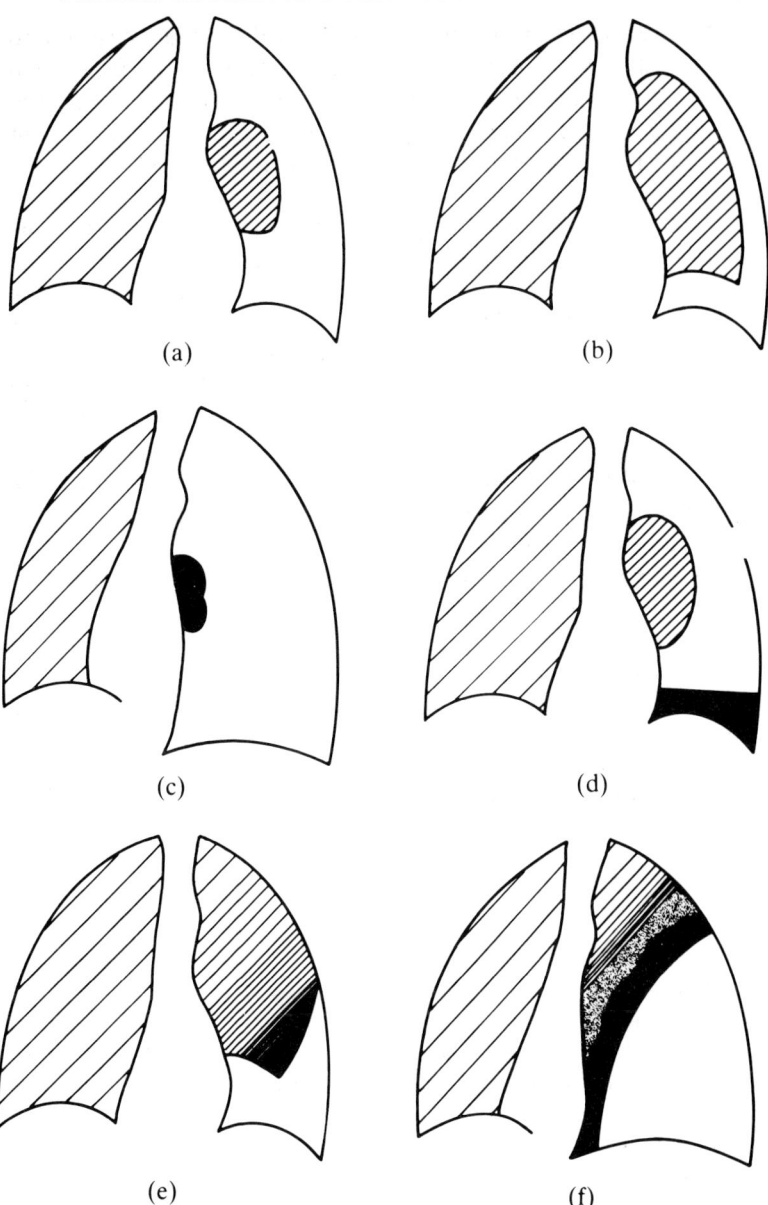

Fig. 12.1 Different types of pneumothorax. (a) Open pneumothorax (breach in visceral pleura), (b) closed pneumothorax, (c) tension pneumothorax (mediastinum displaced to opposite side), (d) traumatic pneumothorax (chest wall injury and blood in pleural cavity), (e) localized pneumothorax, (f) localized tension pneumothorax.

be a predisposing congenital abnormality (Marfan's syndrome). Spontaneous pneumothorax is a serious complication of the respiratory distress syndrome in premature infants and also of adult respiratory distress syndrome (ARDS), especially when treatment with mechanical ventilation employing positive end-expiratory pressure (PEEP) has to be used. It may also complicate a severe attack of asthma at any age.

Fundamental points of diagnosis

The sudden onset of breathlessness often associated with chest pain should always suggest the diagnosis. Clinical confirmation may often be difficult unless the pneumothorax is large. The chest X-ray is vital in diagnosis.

Complications

Tension pneumothorax. The development of a tension pneumothorax may prove fatal even in patients with previously healthy lungs.

Respiratory failure. A shallow pneumothorax occurring in the presence of severe chronic lung disease can rapidly precipitate respiratory failure.

Haemorrhage (haemopneumothorax) is commonly found in traumatic pneumothorax, but blood loss from ruptured pleural adhesions may be considerable in spontaneous pneumothorax.

Infection leading to pyopneumothorax is common in traumatic cases and in patients in whom pneumothorax has been produced by rupture of an abscess cavity into the pleural space.

Pleural thickening may develop in long-standing pneumothoraces, particularly if there is also infection of the pleural space. This may result in failure of re-expansion of the lung unless surgical decortication is performed.

Pulmonary collapse. Bronchial occlusion leading to collapse within an already partially deflated lung can occur in any type of pneumothorax. Sometimes collapse occurs without bronchial obstruction and if it persists for more than a few days it may cause bronchiectasis (p. 46).

Recurrence. It has been estimated that recurrence occurs in some 20% of patients with 'pneumothorax simplex' and in the region of 50% of patients of whom it is a complication of chronic obstructive airways disease.

Mediastinal emphysema is present in many patients with pneumothorax, particularly tension pneumothorax, but is not necessarily a direct complication of the pneumothorax (*see* Mediastinal emphysema). Mediastinal emphysema often occurs without pneumothorax.

Re-expansion pulmonary oedema may rarely complicate rapid re-expansion of the lung after treatment if a large pneumothorax has been present for more than a few days. The cause of this extensive pulmonary shadowing, which looks like pulmonary oedema, is not known.

Clinical findings

Symptoms and signs

The onset is abrupt and often associated with pleuritic-type pain. Central chest discomfort with radiation to the root of the neck is also quite common. Breathlessness is a feature in most patients but may be only noticed on exertion in previously fit individuals. Severe breathlessness is usual in patients with chronic obstructive airways disease or chronic lung disease of any type. Tension pneumothorax is always associated with severe breathlessness and distress. Occasionally there may be a sensation that there is something loose inside the chest, and patients with a left-sided pneumothorax may be aware of a clicking noise.

The clinical signs of a shallow pneumothorax are difficult to elicit, especially in patients with emphysema, or may be overlooked in a patient with asthma (p. 58). Decreased chest expansion, a resonant percussion note and decreased or absent breath sounds are the signs of pneumothorax, but do not differ, except in degree, from those of emphysema. A large pneumothorax is usually easily detectable, especially if the contralateral lung is normal. The percussion note is hyper-resonant and breath sounds absent. In tension pneumothorax there is mediastinal shift to the opposite side (deviation of trachea, cardiac dullness and apex beat) and there may be tachycardia, hypotension, pallor and sweating. The 'coin' sign is of very little value in the diagnosis of pneumothorax.

With left-sided pneumothoraces there may be a 'clicking' sound synchronous with the heart beat. The 'pneumothorax click' can be so loud as to be audible without the aid of a stethoscope. Palpation of the neck may reveal the crepitant evidence of subcutaneous (interstitial) emphysema.

Radiological examination

The chest X-ray is vital in the diagnosis of pneumothorax. It is rarely possible to plan treatment without confirmation of the diagnosis and knowledge of the presence or absence of pleural adhesions. A pneumothorax is recognized by the presence of a clear zone without lung markings between the chest wall and the edge of the lung, which is usually clearly defined. A shallow pneumothorax may, however, be easily missed unless the periphery of the thorax from costophrenic angle to apex is very closely examined. Sometimes a shallow pneumothorax is more easily seen on an X-ray taken on expiration. In large pneumothoraces the lung is seen as a bulbous mass in the centre of the chest at the hilum. The individual lobes of the lung are often clearly outlined. Pleural adhesions are usually easily visible, preventing separation of the lung from the chest wall. Fluid in the pleural space in the presence of pneumothorax has a clear-cut horizontal upper level (fluid level). In tension pneumothorax the mediastinal structures are clearly seen to be displaced to the opposite side.

Investigations

Arterial blood gas analysis must be performed in all patients who develop pneumothorax as a complication of chronic lung disease, since in these patients respiratory failure is frequently precipitated by pneumothorax.

Sputum examination is indicated in all cases where pneumothorax has been produced by the rupture of a cavity into the pleural space. Pyogenic organisms such as *Staphylococcus aureus* should be anticipated in patients with an acute pneumonic illness, but examination for tubercle bacilli must also be made.

Differential diagnosis

Clinically, spontaneous pneumothorax has to be differentiated from other causes of chest pain and breathlessness of sudden onset such as thromboembolic disease, pneumonia and myocardial infarction. When breathlessness is the only symptom the differential diagnostic list is extended to include exacerbations of chronic obstructive airways disease, pleural effusion and bronchial carcinoma. Physical examination is usually sufficient to differentiate pneumothorax from pleural effusion and bronchial carcinoma.

Radiologically large emphysematous bullae sometimes simulate pneumothorax, but usually within bullae there is some pulmonary tissue visible, and a clearly defined lung edge cannot be seen. Occasionally obstructive emphysema and congenital unilateral emphysema may be difficult to differentiate from pneumothorax, especially if the chest X-ray is not technically satisfactory. Overpenetrated chest X-rays often cause confusion, and if this is the case another film should be taken.

Treatment

The major decision in the individual case is whether treatment is necessary. Specific therapy is indicated in:

1 Tension pneumothorax.
2 Pneumothorax causing breathlessness.
3 Bilateral pneumothoraces.
4 Patients who are being mechanically ventilated or being considered for ventilation.
5 Large pneumothorax, i.e. the lung is separated from the chest wall by an air space of one-third or more of the transverse diameter of the hemithorax at the level of the hilum, irrespective of whether or not symptoms are present.
6 When the X-ray shows a large accumulation of pleural fluid.
7 Pneumothorax complicating pulmonary disease such as suppurative pneumonia or tuberculosis, even in the absence of pleural fluid.
8 Recurrent pneumothorax.

Previously fit patients with shallow asymptomatic pneumothoraces do not require treatment, since absorption of the air can be confidently expected within a few days. However, if such patients are managed as out-patients they must be instructed to report to hospital immediately should symptoms develop. Patients living long distances from hospital should be admitted even if specific treatment is not planned.

Specific treatment

Specific treatment of pneumothorax is the removal or drainage of air from the pneumothorax space. Evacuation of air can be attempted using a pneumothorax apparatus, syringe, three-way tap and underwater seal system via a needle introduced into the pleural space, but these methods of treatment have now been mainly superseded by intercostal drainage using an intercostal catheter connected to an underwater seal drain or dry one-way valve (e.g. Heimlich valve). Intercostal catheters are introduced using local anaesthesia and a trocar and cannula (Malecot self-retaining catheter stretched on an introducer) or by the direct insertion of a catheter containing a sharp metal trocar (e.g. Argyle catheter). Generally the second anterior intercostal space is used for intubation, but this site should be avoided for cosmetic reasons in young females, and the fourth or fifth intercostal space just behind the anterior axillary line used instead, providing no adhesions are seen in this site after careful examination of the X-ray. Laterally situated tubes are probably more comfortable because they avoid the pectoral muscles, but have the disadvantages of interfering with arm movement and making the wearing of clothing more difficult.

Initially the intercostal tube should be connected to an underwater seal drain to determine whether there is a persisting pleural leak (open pneumothorax) when air will continue to bubble through the water seal when the patient breathes and coughs. Water seal drainage bottles also allow efficient drainage of fluid or blood from the pleural space. One-way valves allow the patient to be mobile but quickly become blocked if there is much pleural fluid. When large accumulations of pleural fluid are present the patient should be postured according to the site of intercostal intubation to allow drainage.

In the majority of cases, especially in young patients, X-ray will show apposition of the pleural surfaces soon after intercostal drainage has been established. The tube can be removed 24–72 hours after air has stopped bubbling through the water seal. Frequently, however, intercostal tubes become blocked and have to be replaced by new tubes in other sites.

In patients in whom intubation does not achieve re-expansion of the lung in spite of free drainage of air this indicates a large pleural hole allowing air to enter the pleural space at a greater rate than it can be drained through the intercostal catheter. In this situation it is more rational to introduce a second intercostal tube with a separate drainage bottle than to apply suction to the original tube. The use of suction rarely succeeds and when it is used a very powerful suction apparatus has to be employed. If intercostal drainage fails to relieve the pneumothorax which is still 'open', surgical treatment (thoracotomy and removal or oversewing of bullae) may be necessary if the patient's general condition permits this procedure.

Recurrent pneumothorax

Recurrent pneumothorax is treated by pleurodesis or a formal surgical procedure to obliterate the pleural space. Pleurodesis can be achieved by the injection of camphor in oil (10 ml of a 1% solution) into the pleural space, or the insufflation of kaolin. Camphor in oil can be used prior to intercostal intubation under local anaesthesia, but kaolin insufflation should be performed under general anaesthesia whenever possible. Kaolin pleurodesis has proved to be so effective that surgical procedures involving thoracotomy are rarely necessary.

Permanent obliteration of the pleural space can be achieved by parietal pleurectomy or abrasion of the parietal pleura. These procedures obviously involve thoracotomy.

Bilateral pneumothorax

Whenever there is a history of pneumothorax occurring on different sides on separate occasions, or whenever bilateral pneumothoraces occur at the same time, prompt definitive surgical therapy aimed at securing at least one pleural space is indicated.

Tension pneumothorax

Tension pneumothorax is a medical emergency and demands immediate treatment. The insertion of a wide-bore needle or intravenous cannula into the pneumothorax results in the rapid relief of positive pressure within the pneumothorax and dramatic clinical improvement. If the patient is desperately ill and is grossly hypotensive this procedure may have to be performed without X-ray confirmation of the diagnosis. After tension has been relieved the pneumothorax can be treated with relative leisure as outlined above.

High-concentration oxygen therapy

Treatment with very high concentrations of inspired oxygen can increase the rate of absorption of air (mainly nitrogen) from the pneumothorax space by increasing the partial pressure of oxygen in the blood and tissues. However, this treatment is not often used since there is little indication in previously healthy patients, and in patients with chronic obstructive airways disease it may precipitate type II respiratory failure.

Analgesia

The insertion of an intercostal tube using local anaesthesia should be painless, but some patients experience distressing pain at the site of the tube once the anaesthetic has worn off. It is essential to relieve pain as efficiently as possible in order to allow deep breathing and coughing which will aid re-expansion of the lung and prevent complications such as sputum retention. Unless there is a history of severe chronic obstructive airways disease or there is evidence of type II respiratory failure, potent analgesic drugs such as pethidine (100 mg) or morphine (10 mg) should be given.

Physiotherapy

Regular physiotherapy to prevent sputum retention should be routine in all patients. This is of particular importance in those with chronic lung disease. Analgesic drugs should be given an hour or so before physiotherapy to relieve pain and ensure maximum patient co-operation with the physiotherapist.

Prognosis

The prognosis in young previously healthy patients is good although a few will have a recurrence and require pleurodesis. In patients with chronic lung disease of any type the first pneumothorax may be fatal; in survivors, recurrence after medical treatment is common and kaolin pleurodesis or surgical treatment is not always possible, or is hazardous.

MEDIASTINAL EMPHYSEMA

General considerations

Mediastinal emphysema indicates air in the tissues of the mediastinum. Air can escape from alveoli, bronchi or the oesophagus.

Alveolar rupture allowing air to track along peribronchial tissues and enter the mediastinum at the hilum can occur in:

1 Asthma during a severe episode.
2 Any disease causing severe coughing, e.g. whooping cough.
3 During a Valsalva manoeuvre, e.g. straining at stool or during labour.

4   During mechanical ventilation using high inflationary pressure and/or positive end-expiratory pressure (PEEP).

Bronchial rupture may lead to mediastinal emphysema and pneumothorax and can be caused by:

1   Chest injury.
2   Trauma to bronchi at bronchoscopy.

Oesophageal rupture is an extremely serious cause of mediastinal emphysema since it is virtually always associated with acute mediastinitis. The most common site of oesophageal rupture is the left posterolateral wall at its lower end. Oesophageal rupture can be caused by:

1   Chest injury.
2   Trauma to the oesophageal wall during oesophagoscopy, particularly when procedures to dilate strictures are being performed.
3   Vomiting, particularly in alcoholics.
4   Foreign body ingestion, especially animal or fish bones.

Air commonly escapes from the mediastinum into the subcutaneous tissues of the neck but only rarely tracks downwards into retroperitoneal tissues.

Fundamental points of diagnosis

The clinical picture of mediastinal emphysema is usually overshadowed by the precipitating cause such as severe acute asthma or chest trauma. Chest pain and auscultatory findings may be virtually diagnostic, and the diagnosis must always be suggested by the presence of subcutaneous emphysema in the neck. Definitive diagnosis can, however, only be made by chest X-ray.

Complications

Rarely the presence of a large volume of air in the mediastinum can result in compression effects on the heart and major vessels, leading to circulatory collapse. However, hypotension in patients with mediastinal emphysema is much more likely to be due to other complications of the primary cause, e.g. haemopneumothorax or acute mediastinitis.

Clinical findings

Symptoms and signs

Usually there are no specific features of mediastinal emphysema, but occasionally central chest pain similar to ischaemic myocardial pain may be produced. The patient may be aware of swelling and crepitus in the neck caused by subcutaneous emphysema.

A large amount of air in front of the heart may reduce cardiac dullness and heart sounds. Systolic 'clicking' or 'crunching' sounds may be audible over the left sternal edge, particularly when the patient is sitting up. There may be subcutaneous emphysema palpable in the neck. Other clinical abnormalities depend upon the cause of mediastinal emphysema — e.g. lung hyperinflation and rhonchi in asthma, pneumothorax or haemopneumothorax in ruptured bronchus due to chest trauma, left-sided pleural effusion and fever (due to mediastinitis) in ruptured oesophagus.

Radiological examination

Chest X-ray is essential to confirm the diagnosis. The translucency caused by air can be seen outlining the upper mediastinal structures and the heart. The X-ray often also shows air in the tissue planes of the neck (subcutaneous emphysema). Pneumothorax and pleural effusion will be present in some cases.

Investigations

Bronchoscopy or oesophagoscopy may be indicated, depending upon the cause of the mediastinal emphysema.

Differential diagnosis

On clinical grounds myocardial infarction and left-sided pneumothorax may have to be considered, but the diagnosis can usually be established by a chest X-ray. The cause of mediastinal emphysema may, however, be more difficult to determine.

Treatment

Treatment is of the cause and of other complications since specific therapy of mediastinal emphysema is hardly ever necessary. Surgical decompression of the mediastinum by incising the neck above the suprasternal notch has been advocated but is rarely, if ever, indicated. The administration of high concentrations of inspired oxygen can speed up the absorption of air from the tissue planes.

Prognosis

Prognosis depends upon the cause and presence of other complications. Mediastinal emphysema itself is of little clinical importance.

SUMMARY — SPECIAL POINTS OF EMPHASIS

• Tension pneumothorax is a rare but potentially fatal form of pneumothorax.

• Pneumothorax may occur as a complication of chronic lung disease, particularly emphysema.

• A small pneumothorax may be difficult to diagnose clinically, but may cause respiratory failure in patients with chronic obstructive airways disease.

• Sudden onset of breathlessness with or without pleuritic chest pain should always raise the suspicion of spontaneous pneumothorax.

• The chest X-ray is vital in diagnosis and planning of treatment.

• Intercostal intubation and water seal drainage is the most effective method of treatment.

• Pleurodesis is indicated in recurrent pneumothorax and bilateral pneumothoraces.

• Emergency treatment of tension pneumothorax is to release the positive pressure within the pneumothorax by the insertion of a wide-bore needle or intravenous cannula.

• Mediastinal emphysema is caused by damage to alveolar tissue, bronchi or the oesophagus.

• The presence of subcutaneous emphysema in the neck should always raise the suspicion of mediastinal emphysema.

• Mediastinal emphysema itself is of little consequence, but is usually associated with serious disease or injury.

Further reading

Crompton G.K. (1982) Spontaneous pneumothorax. *Hospital Update* **8**, 251–62.
Riordan J.F. (1984) Management of spontaneous pneumothorax. *Brit. med. J.* **289**, 71.

Chapter 13
Occupational lung diseases

Occupational lung disease can be defined as pathological lung changes caused by injurious substances inhaled during the course of employment. The injurious substances can be broadly divided into three main groups:

1 Gases and fumes.
2 Mineral dusts.
3 Organic dusts.

The numerous pathological changes that can be produced in the lungs include: airways obstruction (acute and chronic), allergic alveolitis, pulmonary oedema, pulmonary granulomatosis, pulmonary fibrosis, bronchial carcinoma and pleural mesothelioma.

Pneumoconiosis is the accumulation of dust in the lungs and the tissue reactions to its presence. Dust is defined as an aerosol composed of solid inanimate particles. The most common pneumoconiosis is coalworker's pneumoconiosis (CWP).

The pneumoconioses are occupational lung diseases, but not all occupational lung diseases can be called pneumoconioses.

OCCUPATIONAL AIRWAYS OBSTRUCTION

General considerations

Acute airways obstruction can be induced by a wide variety of potentially hazardous substances encountered in industry. Acute bronchitis can be produced by the inhalation of chemically irritant gases and fumes (Table 13.1) and frequently these substances also cause pulmonary oedema or chemical pneumonia. These effects are directly due to chemical irritation and long-term or repeated exposure may give rise to chronic bronchitis. The occupational causes of airways obstruction are multitudinous and in the future it is likely that many more substances will be identified.

Occupational asthma became a prescribed disease in the U.K. in 1982 — an industrial disease for which disablement benefit can be paid under the Industrial Injuries Scheme. Normally a condition for disablement benefit is that the claimant has been exposed to one of the

Table 13.1 Occupational causes of acute bronchitis, pulmonary oedema or 'pneumonia' and asthma.

Acute bronchitis	Pulmonary oedema or 'pneumonia'		Asthma	
Ammonia	Ammonia	Ozone	Isocyanates	Phenylglycine	Grain dust
Chlorine	Chlorine	Alumina abrasives	Platinum salts	Piperazine	Flour
Sulphur dioxide	Sulphur dioxide	Beryllium oxide	Chrome salts	Spiramycin	Castor bean dust
Sulphur trioxide	Sulphur trioxide	Cadmium oxide	Nickel salts	Proteolytic enzymes	Wood dusts
Vanadium	Phosgene	Osmium tetroxide	Aluminium salts	Phthalic anhydride	Gum acacia
Isocyanates	Oxides of nitrogen	Manganese fumes	Penicillin	Ethylenediamine	Biological washing powders

following seven agents in the course of his work within 10 years preceding his claim:

1   Isocyanates.
2   Platinum salts.
3   Fumes or dusts arising from the manufacture, transport or use of hardening agents (including epoxy resin curing agents) based on phthalic anhydride or tetrachlorophthalic anhydride, trimellitic anhydride or triethylenetetramine.
4   Fumes arising from the use of rosin as a soldering flux.
5   Proteolytic enzymes.
6   Animals or insects used for the purposes of research or education or in laboratories.
7   Dusts arising from the sowing, cultivation, harvesting, drying, handling, milling, transport or storage of barley, oats, rye, wheat or maize, or the handling, milling, transport or storage of meal or flour made therefrom.

Fundamental points of diagnosis

An accurate and detailed history is of fundamental importance in the diagnosis of airways obstruction of occupational cause. Massive exposure to a noxious agent is rarely overlooked, but great care must be taken in patients who have developed hypersensitivity to a substance at work which provokes asthma. In particular it must be appreciated that substances like isocyanates are used in a wide variety of industrial processes.

Complications

Occupational asthma may be severe and potentially fatal. Repeated massive exposure or chronic subacute exposure to chemical irritants can result in chronic obstructive airways disease.

Clinical findings

Symptoms and signs

The clinical findings in patients with occupationally induced airways obstruction are similar to those of acute bronchitis and asthma. Patients who have inhaled irritant chemical substances may also have the features of pulmonary oedema. Accurate diagnosis depends upon the recognition of the history of symptoms coming on after inhalation of a substance at work. Usually symptoms start quickly after exposure, but not always.

Radiological examination

The chest X-ray may be normal or show evidence of lung hyperinflation, pulmonary oedema or 'pneumonia'.

Investigations

Ventilatory function tests will show evidence of airways obstruction. A restrictive defect will also be present in patients who have also developed pulmonary oedema or chemical pneumonia.

An important investigation of possible occupational asthma is the twice-daily, or more frequent, measurement of PEF by the patient with a peak flow gauge. Records of PEF over prolonged periods would be expected to show lower levels on days at work when exposed to the offending agent than at weekends or longer periods of absence from work such as holidays.

Other procedures

When occupational asthma is suspected it may be necessary to prove the diagnosis by performing a provocation test. These tests should always be performed with great care and full facilities for treatment and resuscitation should be readily available since a severe asthmatic episode may be induced even in well-controlled tests.

Differential diagnosis

Airways obstruction developing at work is often due to non-occupational causes and hence all conditions associated with broncho-constriction must be considered.

Treatment

There is no specific treatment for occupationally induced airways obstruction (*see* Treatment of asthma) except for the avoidance of further exposure.

Prognosis

The prognosis depends upon early diagnosis and avoidance of further exposure. Unrecognized disease can lead to chronic irreversible airways obstruction.

Isocyanates can also cause a restrictive pulmonary defect with clinical features similar to those of allergic alveolitis. Failure to recognize this abnormality is likely to result in pulmonary fibrosis.

BYSSINOSIS

Byssinosis is an occupational lung disease characterized by airways obstruction and caused by the inhalation of dusts of cotton, flax or sisal hemp. It usually occurs in workers who have had years of exposure in cotton rooms, blowing rooms or card rooms. The pathogenesis of the disease is not fully understood, but is characterized by symptoms of airways obstruction, usually wheeze and chest tightness, on exposure to the dust after the weekend break. In European countries symptoms develop during the first shift on Mondays and initially are not present on subsequent working days, but return on the first day at work after the next break. As the disease becomes established symptoms are present on the first two days and later more days of each week until the features of the disease are indistinguishable from those of chronic obstructive bronchitis.

Initially, ventilatory function tests show evidence of airways obstruction only at the beginning of each working week. Chest X-ray is normal.

Treatment is by early detection of the disease and removal of workers from the dust hazard. In chronic cases the treatment is the same as that of patients with chronic obstructive bronchitis (*see* p. 37). Smokers have a greater incidence of byssinosis than non-smokers and therefore smoking should be discouraged in all workers at risk.

OCCUPATIONAL PULMONARY OEDEMA

Many of the irritant chemicals which cause acute bronchitis are also capable of producing pulmonary oedema or chemical pneumonia (*see* Table 13.1) which may be severe or fatal. The diagnosis is usually evident because of the history of exposure. The clinical features are similar to those of other causes of pulmonary oedema, except that marked airways obstruction is present in many cases.

Treatment of patients with chemical pulmonary oedema or pneumonia should include corticosteroid therapy as well as high concentrations of oxygen. Diuretic therapy may also be beneficial. A wide-spectrum antibiotic should be given to prevent secondary bacterial infection which is common.

OCCUPATIONAL ALLERGIC ALVEOLITIS

General considerations

The pathogenesis of extrinsic allergic alveolitis is not fully understood, but it seems likely that type III and cell-mediated reactions, together with non-immunological factors, are involved as a response to the inhalation of organic dust. Initially there is oedema of the lungs with a predominantly lymphocytic, and usually also plasma cell, infiltration and thickening of alveolar walls. The oedema subsides over a few days and numerous sarcoid-type non-caseating granulomas develop in the alveolar walls and in the walls of terminal and respiratory bronchioles. The granulomas resolve slowly and are replaced by a substantially lymphocytic inflammatory thickening of the alveolar walls. The end result is irreversible diffuse collagenous fibrosis of alveolar walls, terminal and respiratory bronchioles and also perivascular zones. The hazard is often occupational. The classical example of this disease is farmer's lung caused by the thermophyllic actinomycetes present in the dust of mouldy hay. There are many other causes of occupational extrinsic allergic alveolitis often due to exposure to organic dusts. Some of these are listed in Table 13.2. Other occupations such as vineyard spraying, furriery, coffee manufacture and paprika splitting have also been incriminated in the production of extrinsic allergic alveolitis, but the specific antigens responsible have not been clearly defined. A disease very similar to farmer's lung due to contamination of water in humidifiers or air-conditioning plants (humidifier fever) has been described. As with occupational asthma it is likely that many more causes of extrinsic allergic alveolitis will be discovered in the future.

Not all cases of extrinsic allergic alveolitis are due to occupational exposure to allergens. Indeed the commonest disease of this type in Britain is bird fancier's lung caused by exposure to budgerigars and pigeons. In some the diagnosis may be difficult to make, particularly when birds are kept in the house and exposure to avian allergen is more or less constant.

Therefore, in the investigation of all cases of restrictive pulmonary

Table 13.2 Extrinsic allergic alveolitis.

Disease	Source of antigen	Antigen
Farmer's lung	Mouldy hay	*Micropolyspora faeni* *Thermoactinomyces vulgaris*
Maltworker's lung	Mouldy barley	*Aspergillus clavatus*
Pigeon breeder's lung (bird fancier's lung)	Pigeon droppings and feather bloom Bird droppings and feather bloom	Pigeon droppings and feathers Bird droppings and feathers
Cheese washer's lung	Mouldy cheese	*Penicillium casei*
Mushroom worker's lung	Mushroom compost	*M. faeni and T. vulgaris*
Bagassosis	Mouldy bagasse	*T. sacchari*
Suberosis	Mouldy cork dust	Cork dust
Maple bark stripper's lung	Mouldy maple bark	*Cryptostroma corticale*
Sequoiosis	Mouldy redwood dust	*Aureobasidium pullulans*
Fish worker's lung	Fishmeal, prawns	Fish protein
Wood pulp worker's lung	Mouldy wood pulp	*Alternaria*
	Biological detergent manufacture	*Bacillus subtilis*
Wheat weevil disease	Infected wheat flour	*Sitophilus granarius*
Humidifier fever	Air-conditioner or humidifier	Thermophilic actinomycetes Amoebae

disorders a careful history of non-occupational exposure to potential allergens is important.

A restrictive pulmonary defect, with similar clinical characteristics to extrinsic allergic alveolitis, has been described due to exposure to isocyanates.

Fundamental points of diagnosis

The onset of symptoms and signs some six hours after exposure to the offending substance should suggest a diagnosis of extrinsic allergic alveolitis, but in cases of chronic exposure and, therefore, chronic symptoms the history may not be clear-cut. Moreover, all clinicians must be aware of the possibility of as yet unrecognized causes of extrinsic allergic alveolitis presenting in the future as new manufacturing processes are developed.

Extrinsic allergic alveolitis (including farmer's lung) is now a prescribed occupational disease under the British Industrial Injuries Act and patients with confirmed disease are entitled to benefit.

Complications

The major complication is the development of pulmonary fibrosis and an irreversible restrictive defect. Fibrosis may be present at the time of diagnosis if exposure to the allergen has been chronic, and will certainly develop if exposure is allowed to continue. Extensive pulmonary fibrosis may lead to death from respiratory failure and cor pulmonale.

Clinical findings

Symptoms and signs

Classically there is a delay of approximately six hours after initial exposure to the onset of symptoms. General symptoms of fever and malaise are common, but the major respiratory symptom is breathlessness without wheeze. Unproductive cough, however, also occurs in many patients.

On auscultation end-inspiratory crepitations are audible over all areas of the lung but most easily heard over the lower zones posteriorly.

In the absence of further exposure systemic symptoms subside within a few hours and respiratory symptoms (and X-ray abnormalities) gradually abate in a few days but may persist for two or three weeks. In subacute and chronic cases in which exposure has been prolonged, symptoms, signs and radiological abnormalities may persist for prolonged periods or be permanent.

Radiological examination

In acute cases the chest X-ray may be normal but often shows widespread micronodular shadows more evident in the mid and upper zones. Occasionally the lung fields have a 'ground-glass' appearance or show a diffuse 'honeycomb' picture. In chronic cases the X-ray changes are non-specific. There may be large irregular dense opacities caused by areas of pulmonary fibrosis.

Investigations

White cell count.   In acute cases there is usually a high WCC with a polymorphonuclear leucocytosis. Eosinophilia is not a feature of extrinsic allergic alveolitis.

Serology.   The demonstration of precipitating antibodies in serum to the suspected allergen (e.g. farmer's lung hay (FLH) antigen complex in farmer's lung and *Aspergillus clavatus* antigen in maltworker's lung) is strong confirmatory evidence of the diagnosis, but since some individuals exposed to an allergen develop precipitins without clinical evidence of disease positive serology is not absolutely diagnostic. Also some patients with disease do not have positive serological tests. Fluorescent antibody and radioimmunoassay techniques can also be used to demonstrate specific (IgG) antibodies.

Pulmonary function tests.   Measurement of lung volumes shows a restrictive defect and the carbon monoxide transfer factor is reduced. Ventilatory function tests are normal in uncomplicated cases.

Other procedures

Allergen inhalation provocation tests may have to be performed in the investigation of doubtful cases, and such tests are very important in the investigation of suspected new causes of extrinsic allergic alveolitis. These tests are monitored by regular measurements of body temperature and serial estimations of transfer factor and lung volumes.

Transbronchial lung biopsy and very rarely lung biopsy at

thoracotomy may be necessary to establish the diagnosis. Broncho-alveolar lavage might be of help but can never be diagnostic. Lavage fluid usually contains an excess of lymphocytes.

Differential diagnosis

The differential diagnosis includes pulmonary oedema, atypical pneumonia and fibrosing alveolitis. Sarcoidosis can mimic the radio-logical changes. In chronic cases the many causes of pulmonary fibrosis, including sarcoidosis, have to be considered.

Treatment

Prevention of these diseases can only be achieved by reducing exposure to the allergens either by wearing efficient masks or preferably by reducing the amount of allergen generated in all occupations. Reduction of moisture content of stored hay decreases the allergens responsible for farmer's lung and the Baxter Pneu-Seal mask has been shown to be effective if always worn by farm workers when there is a risk of exposure to dust from mouldy hay.

Whenever possible, patients with extrinsic allergic alveolitis should be advised to change their occupation or job to avoid further exposure to the allergen hazard.

Acute episodes may require treatment with systemic corticosteroids. Prednisolone in a daily dose of 20–40 mg should be given initially with reductions of daily dose by 5 mg at weekly intervals. Patients with type I respiratory failure should be treated with high concentrations of oxygen in the acute stage.

Prognosis

Prognosis is good, providing the diagnosis is made early and further exposure to the allergen can be avoided. Residual impairment is common whenever diagnosis is delayed. If gross pulmonary fibrosis has developed prognosis is poor because of the early development of cor pulmonale and respiratory failure.

THE PNEUMOCONIOSES

The pneumoconioses are caused by the inhalation of mineral dusts, their accumulation in the lungs and the tissue reactions of the lung to their presence. The tissue reactions to different mineral dusts vary considerably (Table 13.3): iron and barium cause little tissue reaction, whereas asbestos can produce considerable fibrosis and also malignant change. A sarcoid-like granulomatous change can be induced by beryllium. There is considerable variation in the ability to clear inhaled dust from the lungs and also in host response to mineral dust retained in the lungs. Hence only a proportion of workers exposed to the same dust hazard develop disease. The commonest pneumoconioses are coalworker's pneumoconiosis, silicosis and asbestosis.

COALWORKER'S PNEUMOCONIOSIS (CWP)

General considerations

CWP results from the retention within the lungs of particles of coal, most of which are less than 5 μm in diameter. Prolonged exposure is necessary for the development of CWP. There is an individual susceptibility and some coal dust is more hazardous than others. CWP is not confined to underground coal face workers. The disease has two main forms, simple and complicated. Complicated CWP is characterized by the development, almost always in the upper lobes, of large areas of fibrosis to which the term progressive massive fibrosis (PMF) is given. The diagnosis of CWP and classification of simple and complicated disease are made by the X-ray appearances.

Fundamental points of diagnosis

The diagnosis of CWP is made from the history of exposure to coal dust, usually in coal miners, taken in conjunction with the X-ray changes.

Table 13.3   Tissue reaction to mineral dust.

Dust	Tissue reaction	Disease
Iron Barium Tin	Little or none	Siderosis Baritosis Stannosis
Coal dust Kaolin Aluminium	Intermediate	Coalworker's pneumoconiosis Kaolinosis Aluminosis
Silica Talc Asbestos	Considerable	Silicosis Talcosis Asbestosis

Complications

Patients with simple CWP may develop PMF if exposure to the dust hazard is allowed to continue. PMF is especially likely to occur in men who have been exposed to relatively high proportions of quartz in the dust they have inhaled. Cavitation of areas of PMF may take place with the production of black sputum (melanoptysis). Extension of PMF causes distortion and destruction of all pulmonary tissues, giving rise to bronchiectasis, pulmonary hypertension and cor pulmonale. Chronic bronchitis and emphysema frequently complicate CWP and in many cases it appears likely that this is due to dust inhalation rather than cigarette smoking alone. However, since many patients with CWP also smoke it is not easy to separate the effects of smoking and coal dust inhalation.

Patients with rheumatoid disease and CWP may develop peripheral round fibrotic nodules in any lobe (Caplan's syndrome). Caplan's syndrome is not confined to CWP since it may develop in patients with rheumatoid disease and other types of pneumoconiosis. Cavitation of peripheral nodules or areas of PMF can occur and may cause pneumothorax. Tuberculosis may develop in patients with CWP and the diagnosis can only be established by examination of sputum since the X-ray changes of PMF often resemble tuberculosis.

Clinical findings

Symptoms and signs

Simple CWP may be asymptomatic but PMF almost invariably causes breathlessness. This may be the only symptom of CWP unless there is melanoptysis. However, many subjects will also complain of the features of associated chronic bronchitis (p. 34).

The clinical signs of CWP are non-specific. No abnormalities are detectable in patients with simple CWP who do not have chronic bronchitis. In other patients there may be signs of chronic bronchitis, emphysema and cor pulmonale. Finger clubbing is not a feature of CWP.

Radiological examination

The diagnosis and categorization of CWP depends upon interpretation of the X-ray abnormalities. Simple CWP is characterized by the presence of small opacities throughout the lung fields. The opacities are graded according to size:

Punctiform = up to 1·5 mm.

Micronodular or miliary = 1·5–3·0 mm.

Nodular = 3·0–10 mm.

The severity of disease is categorized as:

Category 0. Small rounded opacities absent or less profuse than category 1.

Category 1. Small rounded opacities definitely present but few in number.

Category 2. Small rounded opacities numerous. The normal lung markings are still visible.

Category 3. Small rounded opacities very numerous. Normal lung markings are partly or totally obscured.

By using a 12-point scale experts are able to subdivide these categories.

Progressive massive fibrosis is graded into three categories, A, B and C, according to the greatest diameter and extent of the lesions. Standard films of the various categories are used when classifying pneumoconiosis radiologically.

The X-ray may show cavitated PMF or peripheral opacities in patients with rheumatoid disease. The radiological changes of PMF frequently simulate bronchial carcinoma and tuberculosis.

Investigations

Ventilatory function tests show evidence of airways obstruction in the majority of cases because of associated chronic bronchitis and emphysema. There is little or no correlation between VFTs and the X-ray changes of CWP.

Lung volumes may show a restrictive defect because of the 'space-occupying lesion effect' of PMF but frequently because of the combination of emphysema and PMF the results are difficult to interpret.

Transfer factor is reduced mainly because of emphysema.

The ECG may show evidence of right ventricular hypertrophy, and arterial blood gas analysis may show type II respiratory failure in advanced cases.

Serology.   Rheumatoid factor and antinuclear factor may be present in serum, especially in patients with PMF, even in the absence of clinical evidence of a connective tissue disease.

Differential diagnosis

In simple CWP the chest X-ray and history of dust exposure is usually sufficient to clinch the diagnosis, but miliary tuberculosis and sarcoidosis may have to be considered. The development of PMF makes diagnosis more difficult because the radiological features often closely resemble those of bronchial carcinoma and tuberculosis which have to be excluded in many cases. The availability of previous chest X-rays aids diagnosis greatly since PMF rarely changes dramatically in size unless cavitation has occurred.

Treatment

There is no specific treatment for CWP. To avoid development or the progression of PMF all patients should be removed from the dust hazard. All should be encouraged to stop smoking because of the common association of CWP and chronic obstructive airways disease. Treatment for chronic bronchitis should be given as indicated (*see* p. 37), particularly during exacerbations associated with bronchial infection. Regular examination of sputum for tubercle bacilli should be performed and appropriate treatment given if sputum is found to be positive.

Prognosis

The prognosis is good in simple CWP providing it is not associated with significant chronic obstructive airways disease and further exposure to dust hazard can be prevented. The course of PMF is usually relentlessly downhill, cor pulmonale and type II ventilatory failure developing preterminally.

SILICOSIS

Silicosis is caused by the inhalation and retention of dusts containing silica in occupations such as mining, tunnelling, quarrying, stone-dressing, sand blasting, fettling, boiler scaling and in pottery, ceramics and brick manufacture. Silica is potently fibrogenic and can produce widespread pulmonary fibrosis usually much more marked than in coal-worker's pneumoconiosis. Patients with silicosis have a higher incidence of tuberculosis than the general population. As in CWP patients with silicosis often have chronic bronchitis and emphysema.

The diagnosis is suggested by the occupational exposure and the X-ray appearances which are similar to those of coalworker's pneumoconiosis. Cavitation of areas of progressive massive fibrosis may suggest a diagnosis of tuberculosis even though this complication has not occurred. A distinctive radiological feature of silicosis, which is only very rarely seen in other diseases, is 'egg-shell' calcification of enlarged hilar lymph nodes.

Early diagnosis of silicosis is essential since the disease continues to progress even if further dust exposure is avoided. Treatment comprises the prevention of any further exposure to silica and the management of complications as these arise.

ASBESTOSIS

General considerations

Asbestosis is due to inhalation of asbestos dust. It is characterized by pulmonary fibrosis causing a marked restrictive defect. The term asbestosis does not include the other hazards of inhalation, or ingestion, of asbestos — namely pleural lesions (plaques, effusion, diffuse pleural thickening and malignant mesothelioma) bronchial carcinoma and peritoneal mesothelioma (Table 13.4).

It has been estimated that there are at least one thousand different uses for asbestos. Thus exposure may occur in many industries over and above the mining of the compound. Asbestosis can also occur in the neighbourhood of mines and factories as a result of pollution of the atmosphere. Malignant disease can be induced following trivial exposure but the tumour may not develop for 40 years or more. Hence, exposure is likely to be forgotten, even if it was appreciated at the time.

Some of the occupations with obvious exposure to asbestos dust inhalation are: mining, milling and transportation of asbestos,

Table 13.4   Asbestos-related pleuropulmonary problems.

Asbestosis	Diffuse progressive pulmonary fibrosis.
Mesothelioma	Malignant pleural tumour (no known effective treatment).
Pleural plaques	Raised areas of fibrosis in the parietal pleura — usually bilateral.
Pleural calcification	Occurs in the parietal pleural plaques.
Pleural effusion	Can be transient or chronic. N.B. Pleural effusion can also be the presenting feature of mesothelioma.
Diffuse bilateral pleural thickening	Both pleural layers involved by non-specific fibrosis.
Lung cancer	Peripheral adenocarcinoma thought to be asbestos-induced.

manufacture of corrugated sheeting, other building materials and textiles, shipyard workers, pipe laggers and demolition workers.

There are four main types of asbestos: chrysotile, crocidolite (blue asbestos), armosite and anthophyllite. All types are potentially hazardous but chrysotile accounts for about 90% of the world production and hence exposure to this type of asbestos is more likely. Crocidolite probably is responsible for more pleural tumours than other types, possibly because it has a straight elongated particle shape which allows penetration through the lungs to the pleura.

Significant exposure to asbestos increases the risk of lung cancer by a factor of five in both smokers and non-smokers.

Fundamental points of diagnosis

In patients who develop asbestosis there is usually a definite history of exposure, but it must be remembered that carpenters, joiners, electricians and painters may have had exposure by working in the same environment as those working directly with asbestos. The clinical and X-ray picture of pulmonary fibrosis, with other radiological stigmata of asbestos exposure such as calcification of pleural plaques, often suggests the diagnosis even if there is no obvious history of exposure.

Complications

Progressive diffuse pulmonary fibrosis ultimately causes type I respiratory failure and cor pulmonale. Death may be hastened by the development of bronchial carcinoma or pleural mesothelioma. Previously, pulmonary tuberculosis often complicated asbestosis but this complication is not as common as in patients suffering from silicosis.

Clinical findings

Symptoms and signs

There may be no symptoms in the early stages even though the X-ray shows changes of asbestosis or pleural plaques. The prime symptom is breathlessness, which initially is only exertional. Breathlessness at rest, cough and weight loss are common late symptoms.

Due to the diffuse fibrosis crepitations occur at an early stage of the disease but later may be augmented by the development of bronchiectasis due to gross pulmonary distortion by fibrosis. Initially the crepitations are best heard over the lower zones posteriorly. Finger clubbing is a common finding in asbestosis.

The clinical picture may be further complicated by chronic bronchitis (p. 33) and emphysema (p. 42) or the development of bronchial carcinoma (p. 130) or pleural mesothelioma (p. 175).

Radiological examination (Fig. 13.1)

The radiological changes are most marked in the middle and lower zones and may take the form of diffuse mottling or dense streaky shadowing. Often the cardiac outline is blurred and shaggy. In advanced disease the hemidiaphragms are high, indicating shrunken lungs. Pleural plaques, usually bilateral, may be evident in the mid and lower zones, especially when they have become calcified. Calcification in plaques is usually most easily seen on the diaphragmatic surfaces. Oblique X-rays are useful to show pleural plaques not clearly identifiable on conventional PA and lateral films.

There may be radiological evidence of bronchial carcinoma or pleural mesothelioma.

Investigations

Pulmonary function studies show a restrictive defect, even in the absence of symptoms, with impairment of gas transfer and 'small lungs' as judged by lung volume estimation. There may also be evidence of airways obstruction in individual cases.

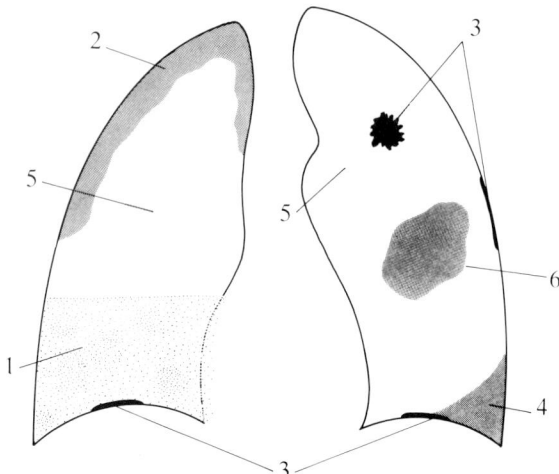

Fig. 13.1 Diagrammatic representation of pleuropulmonary asbestos-related disorders. (1) Asbestosis (pulmonary fibrosis), (2) malignant mesothelioma, (3) pleural calcification, (4) pleural effusion (transient or malignant), (5) pleural thickening (pleural plaques), (6) bronchial carcinoma.

Asbestos bodies.   Asbestos bodies are often present in the sputum, but it must be appreciated that their presence only indicates asbestos inhalation and not necessarily disease. Asbestos bodies are golden yellow, elongated structures with bulbous ends, and are made up of asbestos fibres covered with protein-containing haemosiderin. Asbestos bodies may be recovered in bronchoalveolar lavage fluid which may show an excess of lymphocytes.

Lung biopsy may be necessary in a few cases to establish the diagnosis. It may not be possible to obtain an adequate specimen of lung for histological diagnosis by transbronchial biopsy, but since bronchoscopy is often necessary to exclude or confirm the presence of co-existing bronchial carcinoma transbronchial lung biopsy should always be performed before resorting to formal open thoracotomy biopsy.

Differential diagnosis

The differential diagnosis includes all causes of diffuse pulmonary fibrosis including fibrosing alveolitis and sarcoidosis. It is often difficult to distinguish cryptogenic fibrosing alveolitis from asbestosis.

Treatment

There is no specific treatment for asbestosis. Patients must avoid further exposure. The evidence that corticosteroids are of value is unconvincing, but a therapeutic trial is justified in all cases except those with very advanced disease. This is particularly important if the alternative diagnoses of fibrosing alveolitis and sarcoidosis have not been firmly excluded. Care must be taken, however, before giving corticosteroids to ensure that tuberculosis has not developed as a complication.

Treatment of cor pulmonale and respiratory failure becomes necessary as pulmonary fibrosis advances. Type I respiratory failure develops relatively early and eventually requires treatment with oxygen (p. 82).

Whenever bronchial carcinoma is also diagnosed in a patient with asbestosis the outlook is usually hopeless, since the disordered pulmonary function produced by asbestosis usually precludes definitive treatment, particularly surgical resection.

Prognosis

The vast majority of cases of asbestosis relentlessly progress to death from cor pulmonale and respiratory failure. If bronchial carcinoma or pleural mesothelioma also develop the prognosis is worse.

BERYLLIOSIS

Berylliosis is caused by the inhalation of beryllium compounds. It is described separately because unlike other pneumoconioses in its chronic form it causes granuloma formation as well as pulmonary fibrosis.

Beryllium compounds are not used as extensively in industrial processes as previously, but still have a place in electronics, aeroengine manufacture and atomic reactors.

Acute berylliosis is uncommon, but an acute chemical pneumonia or pulmonary oedema can develop within a few weeks of exposure. Most cases recover spontaneously leaving a variable degree of pulmonary fibrosis, but in some fulminating cases the disease can prove fatal. Corticosteroid therapy should be given to all patients as soon as the diagnosis is established.

Chronic berylliosis is also very rare, but is a unique pneumoconiosis because it causes generalized sarcoid-like granulomatous inflammation associated with fibrosis. Exposure to beryllium does not have to be massive or prolonged and there may be a latent period of 10 years or so before the pulmonary changes develop. The main symptom is breathlessness and pulmonary function studies show a restrictive defect. The chest X-ray initially shows micronodular shadowing throughout both lung fields and later coarser nodulation and hilar enlargement. The course of the disease is similar to pulmonary sarcoidosis, progression occurring in some cases. Treatment with prednisolone should be given as soon as the diagnosis has been established.

SUMMARY — SPECIAL POINTS OF EMPHASIS

• Occupational lung diseases may be caused by inhalation of gases and fumes, mineral dusts and organic dusts.

• Airways obstruction, pulmonary oedema, allergic alveolitis, pulmonary granulomatosis, pulmonary fibrosis, bronchial carcinoma and pleural mesothelioma may result from industrial exposure to noxious substances.

• Occupational asthma is a consequence of sensitization to an agent which is first encountered at work.

• Isocyanates are widely used compounds which may cause asthma and also, less commonly, a restrictive pulmonary defect.

• Farmer's lung is a characteristic example of occupational extrinsic allergic alveolitis but the most common type of this disease in Britain is bird fancier's lung.

• Extrinsic allergic alveolitis classically results in symptoms developing some six hours after exposure to the allergen but where exposure is chronic the diagnosis may be overlooked.

• Extrinsic allergic alveolitis causes a restrictive pulmonary defect, the main symptom of which is breathlessness without wheeze.

• Pulmonary fibrosis is a consequence of continued exposure to allergen in patients with extrinsic allergic alveolitis.

• Pneumoconiosis is defined as the accumulation of dust (inanimate particles) in the lungs and the tissue reactions to its presence.

• The commonest pneumoconiosis is coalworker's pneumoconiosis.

- Coalworker's pneumoconiosis has two main forms — simple and complicated.

- Complicated coalworker's pneumoconiosis is characterized by the development of progressive massive fibrosis.

- Coalworker's pneumoconiosis is frequently associated with chronic bronchitis and emphysema.

- Silica dust (silicosis) causes more fibrosis than coal dust.

- Patients with silicosis have a greater chance of developing pulmonary tuberculosis than patients with normal lungs.

- Asbestosis refers to pulmonary fibrosis caused by asbestos inhalation. Asbestos can also cause pleural plaques, pleural effusion, pleural calcification, pleural mesothelioma and bronchial carcinoma.

- Asbestos bodies in the sputum simply indicate inhalation of asbestos fibres and not necessarily the presence of disease.

- Patients with any form of pneumoconiosis must be advised to avoid further exposure to the dust.

Further reading

Department of Health and Social Security NI 226 (1979) *Pneumoconiosis and related occupational diseases: Notes on Diagnosis and Claims for Industrial Injuries Scheme Benefits.* London: DHSS.
Department of Health and Social Security NI 238 (1982) *Clinical Notes on Occupational Asthma: a Disease Prescribed under the Industrial Injuries Scheme.* London: DHSS.
Gee G.L., Morgan K.C. & Brooks S.M. (1983) *Occupational Lung Disease.* New York: Raven Press.
Morgan W.K.C. & Seaton A. (1984) *Occupational Lung Diseases*, 2nd Edition. Philadelphia: W.B. Saunders Co.
Parkes W.R. (1984) *Occupational Lung Disorders.* London: Butterworth.
Weil H. & Turner–Warwick M. (Eds.) (1981) *Lung Biology in Health and Disease.* Vol. 18 *Occupational Lung Diseases.* New York: Marcel Dekker Inc.

Chapter 14
Cryptogenic fibrosing alveolitis

Synonyms for this disease include diffuse intersitial pulmonary fibrosis, idiopathic interstitial pulmonary fibrosis, idiopathic fibrosing alveolitis, Hamman–Rich syndrome, desquamative interstitial pneumonia, giant cell interstitial pneumonia.

General considerations

Cryptogenic fibrosing alveolitis (CFA) is a disease, or group of diseases, of unknown aetiology pathologically characterized by cellular infiltration and thickening of alveolar walls in the presence of large mononuclear cells in alveolar spaces. There is a variable degree of fibrosis and in most cases progressive fibrosis occurs. It is known that whatever the cause the alveolar macrophages and neutrophils are 'activated' and produce cellular chemotactic and activating factors. It has been suggested that the release of oxidants from neutrophils, and to a lesser extent eosinophils and alveolar macrophages, is one of the mechanisms of tissue injury. Alveolar macrophages are probably involved in the production of fibrosis by their release of fibronectin and alveolar macrophage–derived growth factor. In some patients with CFA there may be evidence of disorders of other systems, such as polyarthritis, rheumatoid disease, systemic lupus erythematosus, systemic sclerosis, myositis, chronic active hepatitis, Sjögren's syndrome, Raynaud's phenomenon, digital vasculitis, ulcerative colitis, thyroid disease, pernicious anaemia, myelosclerosis, folic acid deficiency, adult coeliac disease, and renal tubular acidosis. Although the list of associated diseases is impressive and may suggest that the pulmonary lesion is the result of an autoimmune reaction, the majority of cases of CFA present without clinical or immunological evidence of disease in other systems. The association between CFA and connective tissue disorders such as rheumatoid disease ('rheumatoid lung') is, however, accepted.

The disease can develop at all ages and in both sexes. The majority of patients are middle-aged or elderly. Rarely it can affect more than one member of a family.

CFA must be distinguished from the many other causes of diffuse pulmonary fibrosis which include:

1 Extrinsic allergic alveolitis.
2 Chronic pulmonary oedema.
3 Sarcoidosis.
4 'Histiocytosis X' diseases.
5 Beryllium disease.
6 Asbestosis and other pneumoconioses.
7 Organizing pneumonias.
8 Lung disease induced by various drugs:

Busulphan	Vincristine
Hexamethonium	Nitrofurantoin
Bleomycin	Sulphasalazine
Methotrexate	Mecamylamine
Chlorambucil	Pentolinium
Cyclophosphamide	Gold salts
Melphalan	

Fundamental points of diagnosis

Diagnosis in the majority of cases can be made from the characteristic history of progressive breathlessness without wheeze or cough, together with the clinical findings of widespread end-inspiratory crepitations, and usually finger clubbing, in the absence of asbestos exposure or any other cause of diffuse pulmonary fibrosis.

Complications

Progressive deterioration with early development of type I respiratory failure is the rule. There is probably an increased incidence of bronchial carcinoma.

Clinical findings

Symptoms and signs

Progressive breathlessness, initially noticed only on exertion, is the main symptom. Cough may develop as a late manifestation, but wheeze is not a feature.

Finger clubbing, which is frequently gross and may be associated with X-ray evidence of hypertrophic pulmonary osteoarthropathy, occurs in some 60% of cases. Chest expansion is reduced and respiratory frequency increased. Widespread loud crepitations ('crackling crepitations') are audible over all lung areas but usually best heard over the lower zones posteriorly and laterally. The crepitations are usually limited to the end of inspiration and do not disappear after coughing. In cases with extensive fibrosis bronchial breathing may occasionally develop. Central cyanosis is evident in advanced disease and there may also be signs of cor pulmonale.

Radiological examination

The chest X-ray shows bilateral small irregular shadows, most evident in the lower zones. In advanced disease the lungs are small and may show 'honeycombing'. Pleural abnormalities are uncommon (cf. asbestosis).

Investigations

Investigations are required not only to establish a diagnosis and to assess the severity of the disease, but also as appropriate to exclude possible associated conditions.

Lung volumes.   The vital capacity is reduced and the total lung capacity is low (restrictive defect).

Carbon monoxide transfer (or diffusing capacity) is much reduced.

Ventilatory function tests show no evidence of airways obstruction and the FEV_1/FVC ratio may be increased.

Measurements of lung compliance may confirm a picture of 'stiff lungs'.

Arterial blood gas analysis shows type I respiratory failure precipitated or made worse by exercise.

Bronchoalveolar lavage (BAL).   The differential cell count of BAL fluid reflects the altered cellular populations found in specimens obtained by open-lung biopsy. Active fibrosing alveolitis is characterized by the discovery of raised numbers of neutrophils and eosinophils. A single BAL differential cell count may be of value in assessing the activity of disease and thereby provide information about prognosis and the need to give treatment. Serial lavages may be helpful in assessing response to treatment.

Transbronchial lung biopsy. Since the biopsy specimens obtained by this technique are tiny and have a substantial sampling error transbronchial lung biopsy is of limited value in CFA.

Gallium-67 scanning. Gallium-67 is taken up by the inflammatory cells in CFA and increased counts over the lungs correlates reasonably well with cellular histology. Gallium-67 lung scans in conjunction with bronchoalveolar lavage may be helpful in assessing disease activity and monitoring therapy.

Immunological tests. Total serum globulins may be raised with increases in immunoglobulins, IgG, IgM and IgA. Antinuclear factor, rheumatoid factor, non-organ specific complement fixing antibodies, mitochondrial antibodies and smooth muscle antibodies may be present in the blood of some patients.

Other procedures

Occasionally lung biopsy may be necessary in atypical cases.

Differential diagnosis

The differential diagnosis includes all the causes of diffuse pulmonary fibrosis (*see above*).

Treatment

The majority of patients do not respond well to treatment. Just over 50% of patients are subjectively improved by corticosteroid therapy, but in only about 20% is there objective improvement in pulmonary function tests and/or chest X-ray. Nevertheless, the life expectancy in patients who only subjectively improve is longer than that of non-responders. Perhaps bronchoalveolar lavage and gallium-67 scanning will prove to be more sensitive determinants of response. The treatments available are corticosteroids and immunosuppressive drugs. Prednisolone is the mainstay of treatment, but azathioprine or cyclophosphamide can be used in a steroid-sparing role.

Selection of patients for treatment

A trial of prednisolone therapy is indicated in most patients with progressive disease. In some elderly patients the disease is relatively benign and either progresses very slowly or becomes 'burnt out'. In these patients treatment may be more hazardous than the disease. However, in the majority of cases progression is observed by serial measurements of lung volumes and transfer factor. The response to prednisolone therapy is unpredictable but tends to be better in acute or subacute cases than in patients with chronic disease. Since it is important to avoid ineffective long-term corticosteroid therapy, a formal therapeutic trial of prednisolone must be undertaken in all patients in whom there is an indication for treatment.

Assessment of response to prednisolone

1.   Baseline lung volumes, transfer factor, chest X-ray, and when possible bronchoalveolar lavage and gallium-67 scan.
2.   Treatment with prednisolone in a daily dose of 40–60 mg for six to eight weeks.
3.   Assessment of response by repeat measurements of lung volumes and transfer factor and also X-ray, bronchoalveolar lavage and gallium-67 scan.
4.   If no improvement prednisolone treatment should be withdrawn rapidly, i.e. immediate reduction to 20 mg daily and thereafter withdrawal of therapy over a few weeks. If objective evidence of improvement is demonstrated gradual reductions to a maintenance dose of 10 or 12·5 mg daily should be made. Long-term treatment must be with the smallest dose of prednisolone necessary to control the disease. In most cases, however, it is not possible to reduce the daily dose of prednisolone to much below 10 mg even when azathioprine is added. Serial measurements of lung volumes and transfer factor are essential to assess long-term therapy. The chest X-ray is a less reliable monitor of progress.

Immunosuppressive drugs may be tried in patients in whom the disease has been found to be corticosteroid unresponsive, or in patients in whom there is a contraindication to corticosteroid therapy.

Prognosis

The overall prognosis of CFA is poor. Young patients with acute disease tend to respond better to treatment than the majority of older patients. It has been suggested that a bronchoalveolar lavage neutrophil count of 10% or more carries a poor prognosis. Seventy-five per cent of patients die within eight years of diagnosis.

SUMMARY — SPECIAL POINTS OF EMPHASIS

• CFA is a disease, or group of diseases, of unknown aetiology characterized by progressive alveolar fibrosis.

• A few patients with CFA have clinical or immunological evidence of connective tissue disease, e.g. 'rheumatoid lung'.

• CFA has to be distinguished from the many causes of pulmonary fibrosis.

• The classical symptom is progressive breathlessness; crepitations are almost invariably audible on auscultation and some 60% of patients have finger clubbing.

• Type I respiratory failure develops in most cases. There is probably an increased risk of bronchial carcinoma.

• Pulmonary function studies show a restrictive defect.

• Bronchoalveolar lavage, differential cell counts and gallium-67 lung scans may be of value in assessing disease activity and response to treatment.

• Only a few patients respond to treatment with prednisolone, usually those with relatively acute disease, but a formal trial of treatment is necessary in most.

• 75% of patients are dead within eight years of diagnosis.

Further reading

Johnson A.J. (1982) Cryptogenic fibrosing alveolitis. *Hospital Update* **8**, 1085–98.
Simmons D.H. (Ed.) (1981) *Current Pulmonology, Vol. 3*. New York: John Wiley & Sons.
Turner-Warwick M. (1978) *Immunology of the Lung*. London: Edward Arnold.

Chapter 15
Pulmonary thromboembolic disease

Pulmonary thromboembolic disease has replaced pneumonia as the most common lung disease in hospital practice.

Pulmonary embolism is said to have occurred when a thrombus lodges in the pulmonary artery or one of its branches.

Pulmonary infarction is the term used to describe the pathological changes which may take place in the lungs after occlusion of a branch of the pulmonary artery.

The most common sources of emboli are the veins of the lower limbs and pelvis, but thrombosis in any vein and intracardiac thrombosis can give rise to pulmonary embolism. The incidence of venous thrombosis and pulmonary embolism increases with age and the majority of fatal episodes of this disease occur in patients over the age of 50. Thromboembolic disease may be spontaneous, but often a predisposing cause can be defined. Conditions resulting in venous stasis classically lead to venous thrombosis, but abnormalities of blood coagulability and perhaps fibrinolysis aid the formation of thrombi in some cases. Some of the common predisposing factors are:

1   Age.
2   Surgical operations.
3   Immobility from any cause, including bed rest or travel.
4   Cardiac disorders.
5   Malignant disease.
6   Pregnancy.
7   The contraceptive pill.
8   Blood dyscrasias, particularly thrombocythaemia.
9   Obesity.
10 Trauma.
11 Dehydration.
12 Infections and malnutrition.

Pulmonary thromboembolic disease can be conveniently divided into three clinical types:

(i)   Massive pulmonary embolism.
(ii) Pulmonary infarction.
(iii) Thromboembolic pulmonary hypertension.

It must be stressed, however, that different clinical types of disease may be present in the same patient, and in some patients the clinical picture does not readily fit into one of these arbitrary clinical syndromes.

MASSIVE PULMONARY EMBOLISM

Fundamental points of diagnosis

Patients who develop massive pulmonary embolism may have previously had the clinical features of pulmonary infarction which may not have been recognized. Obvious deep vein thrombosis is present in a minority of patients. The sudden onset of catastrophic disease (*see below*) readily suggests the diagnosis when pulmonary embolism is anticipated after major surgery, or in the presence of clinically diagnosed deep vein thrombosis. However, massive pulmonary embolism must be considered in any patient who becomes suddenly ill with hypotension, central chest pain, faintness and breathlessness. The most fundamental point of diagnosis is the awareness of the possibility of massive pulmonary embolism, even if the circumstances are not classical and the clinical picture is not typical.

Complications

Pulmonary infarction may subsequently develop in some patients. The major complication of massive pulmonary embolism is sudden death, which unfortunately may be its presentation.

Clinical findings

Symptoms and signs

Many patients developing massive pulmonary embolism can in retrospect be seen to have had an unrecognized episode of minor embolism, often leading to infarction — the so-called 'herald infarct'. There may be prodromal features of low-grade pyrexia, haemoptysis and pleuritic pain.

The onset of symptoms is characteristically sudden. Severe breathlessness, central chest pain and a feeling of impending doom are typical, but in some patients the presentation may be with faintness, dizziness or loss of consciousness accompanied by hyperventilation. Pleuritic chest pain and haemoptysis are not features of massive embolism, but may be evidence of previous thromboembolic episodes which have caused pulmonary infarction.

Air hunger, cyanosis, shock, tachycardia and a low blood pressure are constant clinical features, but there may be no abnormalities on examination of the lungs, unless previous pulmonary infarction has occurred. Very occasionally pulmonary embolism induces bronchospasm. A gallop rhythm may be heard on auscultation of the heart but rarely is there clinical evidence of pulmonary hypertension. The jugular venous pressure is usually elevated and other signs of right heart failure may ensue.

Radiological examination

The radiological changes of massive pulmonary embolism are paucity of vascular markings and enlargement of the main pulmonary artery and right ventricle. However, the chest X-ray is frequently of little diagnostic value, since it is difficult to obtain technically good X-rays in these very ill patients and the changes are rarely detected on 'portable' chest X-rays. Changes of previous pulmonary infarction (the 'herald infarct') may be more valuable.

Lung scan.   The perfusion lung scan is grossly abnormal. It may show major defects of perfusion or total lack of perfusion of one lung. However, the lung scan is of little help in diagnosis in patients with co-existing bronchopulmonary or cardiac disease and it is often technically difficult to obtain a satisfactory scan in ill patients. A grossly abnormal scan together with an X-ray showing normal lung fields, in a patient suspected of having a massive pulmonary embolism, is of great value. Ventilation/perfusion scans can enhance the accuracy of scanning in patients with cardiorespiratory disease, but cannot readily be performed in all hospitals.

Pulmonary angiography.   The pulmonary angiogram is the single investigation which can confirm the diagnosis of massive pulmonary embolism. Massive defects of perfusion and sometimes the centrally situated embolism itself are shown by angiography. A normal pulmonary angiogram excludes the diagnosis. If angiography confirms massive embolism the pulmonary artery catheter should be left in position to monitor pressure and to provide a convenient, though not essential, route for infusion of thrombolytic treatment.

Investigations

Electrocardiogram. The ECG may be helpful in diagnosis when it shows evidence of acute right ventricular strain or acute cor pulmonale, but often it is normal and on occasions suggests myocardial infarction.

Blood tests. There are no haematological or biochemical investigations which confirm a massive pulmonary embolism. The measurement of fibrinogen degradation products (FDPs) may be of some value if the patient's normal levels are known, since a transient rise of FDPs accompanies most embolic episodes.

Arterial blood gas analysis. Shows type I respiratory failure. Profound hypoxaemia, which is not readily reversed by the administration of high concentrations of oxygen, invariably results from massive pulmonary embolism. The carbon dioxide tension is low due to alveolar hyperventilation.

Differential diagnosis

Myocardial infarction is most often the alternative diagnosis (Table 15.1). The central chest pain of massive embolism is due to myocardial ischaemia and initially at least the ECG may be misleading. Serum enzymes may confirm myocardial damage, but it must be remembered that pulmonary embolism can lead to myocardial infarction. Spontaneous pneumothorax and massive pulmonary collapse can usually be differentiated by the clinical features and the chest X-ray.

Table 15.1 Conditions pulmonary thromboembolic disease often simulates.

Bronchopulmonary	
Pneumonia	Similar X-ray shadowing, leucocytosis, pyrexia, pleuritic pain.
Asthma	Embolism occasionally induces bronchoconstriction.
Lung abscess	Infection of a pulmonary infarct rapidly results in cavitation.
Tuberculosis	Cavitation of uncommonly situated infarcts in the upper lobes can simulate tuberculosis.
Carcinoma	Radiographically infarcts can look like tumours. (Malignant disease predisposes to thromboembolic disease.)

Table 15.1 *Continued*

Circulatory disorders	
Myocardial infarction	Central chest pain of massive embolism caused by underperfusion of coronary arteries.
Acute right heart failure	Readily precipitated by thromboembolic disease in patients with pre-existing cardiorespiratory problems.
Congestive cardiac failure	'Refractory' cardiac failure often precipitated by thromboembolism in patients with heart disease.
Dysrhythmias	Pulmonary embolism often causes atrial fibrillation and other dysrhythmias but is seldom considered as a cause of arrhythmia.
Cardiac asthma	Thromboembolism as well as pulmonary oedema can cause nocturnal breathlessness and wheeze.
Neurological disorders	
Loss of consciousness	Unconsciousness can be induced in elderly patients by embolism without much other evidence of circulatory disturbance.
Dizziness	A frequent symptom of hypotension induced by pulmonary embolism.
Stroke	Systemic hypotension caused by pulmonary embolism can cause localized neurological deficit in patients with pre-existing cerebral atheroma.
Others	
Septicaemic shock ⎫ Hypovolaemic shock ⎭	Hypotension caused by massive pulmonary embolism in the post-operative patient is often difficult to distinguish from blood loss and septicaemia.
Acute abdominal emergencies	Pulmonary infarction associated with diaphragmatic pleurisy often simulates acute abdominal emergencies such as perforated peptic ulcer and acute cholecystitis.

Treatment

Massive pulmonary embolism is one of the few genuine acute medical emergencies. The majority of deaths occur within two hours, and hence survival can be anticipated if initial resuscitative measures are effective. The choice of treatment theoretically should depend upon the severity of circulatory collapse produced by the embolic event, but in practice is more often governed by the immediate availability of trained personnel and facilities. The treatments available are:

1   External cardiac massage.
2   Embolectomy.
3   Thrombolytic therapy.
4   Heparin.
Plus supportive treatment.

1   *External cardiac massage* must always be performed in unconscious patients. Theoretically cardiac massage can break up and dislodge large centrally situated emboli resulting in more peripheral vascular occlusion and an improved haemodynamic state.

2   *Embolectomy* is rarely performed, since ideally the diagnosis should be confirmed by angiography and the operation carried out with cardio-pulmonary bypass. Emergency embolectomy without cardiopulmonary bypass is rarely successful. The successful removal of embolus from the pulmonary artery by a suction catheter inserted via a femoral vein has been reported.

3   *Thrombolytic therapy.*   Lysis of emboli with streptokinase can achieve rapid clinical improvement, but complications such as haemorrhage and allergic reactions are relatively common, and expert haematological monitoring of treatment is essential. Ideally streptokinase should only be used after pulmonary angiography has been employed to confirm the diagnosis and to assess the degree of pulmonary vascular occlusion. The dose is 250 000 units over 30 minutes followed by 100 000 units an hour for 24 hours. Hydrocortisone should also be given as prophylaxis against allergic reactions.

4   *Heparin.*   Most patients with massive pulmonary embolism are treated with heparin and this drug should be given intravenously in a dose of 10 000 to 15 000 units as soon as the clinical diagnosis is made. Slow intravenous infusion of heparin can then be continued when indicated and the rate monitored by regular laboratory coagulation tests of thrombin time. Treatment with heparin can produce dramatic improvement, which is unlikely to be due simply to its anticoagulant

properties. The suppression of release of vasoactive and perhaps bronchoconstrictor substances from platelets probably partially explains the rapid therapeutic effects of heparin.

In practice there are often no clear-cut indications for the choice of embolectomy, streptokinase or heparin. If pulmonary angiography has been performed and facilities exist to allow a choice of treatment a reduction of pulmonary perfusion of 75% or more is an indication for embolectomy. The choice between streptokinase and heparin is less clear-cut, but thrombolytic therapy has been shown to accelerate angiographic resolution and decrease pulmonary artery pressure more rapidly than treatment with heparin.

Supportive therapy

Supportive therapy is essential in all patients to relieve pain and apprehension, to combat hypoxaemia and to maintain or improve systemic blood pressure. Morphine (10–15 mg i.v.) or diamorphine (5–10 mg i.v.) should be given to all distressed conscious patients. There is no risk of precipitating carbon dioxide retention, unless there is co-existing chronic obstructive airways disease. Indeed, suppression of the extreme degree of hyperventilation induced by pulmonary embolism can in itself improve the clinical state.

Profound hypoxaemia is present in all cases and the administration of high concentrations of oxygen is necessary to improve arterial oxygenation.

Severe hypotension indicates occlusion of a very large proportion of the pulmonary arterial circulation and hence carries a poor prognosis unless embolectomy can be performed or thrombolytic therapy given. Isoprenaline by intravenous infusion (0·5–10 $\mu g/min$) may maintain blood pressure pending more definitive therapy.

Prognosis

Patients who survive for 6–12 hours after massive pulmonary embolism usually make a complete recovery. The availability of facilities for emergency embolectomy and streptokinase therapy in some centres has improved the initial prognosis. However, prevention of venous thromboembolism by prophylactic anticoagulant treatment in patients at risk and the earlier recognition and treatment of deep vein thrombosis and 'herald' pulmonary infarction is much more likely to reduce mortality from this disease than any improvement in treatment.

PULMONARY INFARCTION

Fundamental points of diagnosis

Pulmonary infarction has no unique symptoms, signs or investigation findings during life. Awareness of the possibility that pulmonary infarction can simulate other pulmonary diseases, notably pneumonia, is of vital importance if the diagnosis is to be made at an early stage. Rarely is there clinical evidence of deep vein thrombosis in association with pleuritic pain, haemoptysis and breathlessness. This 'full house' of clinical abnormalities does not occur in the majority of patients since deep vein thrombosis is often silent and pulmonary infarction does not always produce the classical symptoms. A combination of haemoptysis and pleuritic pain should always suggest pulmonary infarction. The chest X-ray changes are sometimes suggestive but never diagnostic.

Complications

Pleural effusions are common; however, most are small and do not require specific treatment. Occasionally large effusions develop in previously healthy patients but massive effusions most often complicate pulmonary infarction in patients with heart disease (e.g. mitral stenosis). The fluid is usually serous but may be haemorrhagic, and may contain large numbers of eosinophils.

Infection of a pulmonary infarct is usually from a bronchial source. Only rarely is the embolus itself infected (septic embolism). Infection can rapidly lead to lung abscess, bronchopleural fistula and empyema.

Spontaneous pneumothorax occurs rarely.

Pulmonary collapse occurs when a large bronchus becomes occluded by blood clot, usually in patients coughing up copious quantities of blood, and especially when coughing is restricted by pleuritic pain.

Failure to recognize and treat pulmonary infarction may allow massive pulmonary embolism or thromboembolic pulmonary hypertension to develop.

Clinical findings

Symptoms and signs

There may be an initial period suggesting a fairly large embolism such as a dizzy turn, transient central chest pain or a sudden attack of breathlessness. The most frequent symptom of pulmonary infarction is pleuritic pain not preceded by an upper respiratory tract infection or non-specific symptoms of pyrexia.

Haemoptysis is the next most common symptom. It may be massive and is not associated, initially at least, with purulent sputum.

Breathlessness is seldom severe and most often is due to pleuritic pain.

CLINICAL SIGNS

Low-grade pyrexia is common and occasionally fever can be high (39°C) in patients with non-infected infarcts. A high fever can cause rigors, but fever with rigors is uncommon in pulmonary infarction compared with pneumonia. The degree of tachycardia is usually out of proportion to the pyrexia. Physical signs are similar to those found in pneumonia. However, bilateral signs are more common in infarction than in infection. Pleural friction rubs are quite common and may be present in patients without pleuritic pain. Signs of consolidation, pulmonary collapse or effusion may be present, but often the only abnormal finding is the presence of inspiratory crepitations. Signs produced by a raised hemidiaphragm may be mistaken for those of pleural effusion or pulmonary collapse. Chest wall tenderness at the site of pleuritic pain is often present but this is not a specific feature of pulmonary infarction.

Radiological examination

The chest X-ray abnormalities suggestive of pulmonary infarction are (Fig. 15.1):

The abnormalities are often bilateral. Pleural and pulmonary shadows are usually in the lower zones.

1 Linear shadows which are often large and do not conform to the bronchopulmonary segmental architecture are much more often associated with pulmonary infarction than any other pulmonary disease. The linear opacities are often referred to as 'plate atelectasis'.
2 Elevation of one hemidiaphragm is common.
3 Pulmonary opacities, most of which are in the lower lobes, are rarely truly segmental or lobar in outline compared with pneumonic consolidation. Round, fairly well circumscribed shadows can occur but the classical triangular-shaped opacity, with its base on the pleural surface, is rare.
4 Pleural effusion(s).

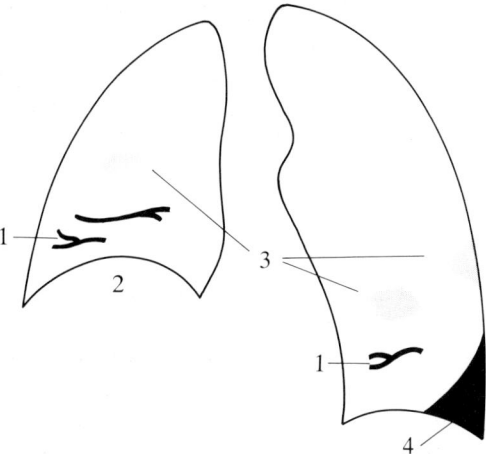

Fig. 15.1   Diagrammatic representation of the X-ray abnormalities which should arouse the suspicion of pulmonary infarction. (1) Lower zone linear shadows, (2) elevated hemidiaphragm, (3) bilateral hazy non-segmental pulmonary shadows, (4) pleural effusion(s).

Screening of a raised hemidiaphragm may reveal paradoxical movement. The mechanism of diaphragmatic paralysis in pulmonary infarction is not understood.

Perfusion lung scan.   The lung scan in pulmonary infarction typically shows much more gross abnormalities of perfusion than is suggested by the plain X-ray. However, interpretation of the lung scan can be difficult, particularly in patients with co-existing airways disease or heart disease. Hence, this investigation is of greatest value in patients whose cardiorespiratory systems were normal before the suspected pulmonary embolic event. Nevertheless this method remains the mainstay of diagnosis. Scanning accuracy can be improved by the combined ventilation/perfusion scan, particularly in patients with pre-existing cardiopulmonary disease. A negative scan result is of great value, as is a clearly positive scan. The scan showing equivocal abnormalities may act as an invaluable baseline for follow-up examination. In pneumonia the scan abnormalities rarely exceed those seen on the chest X-ray.

A normal X-ray does not exclude a diagnosis of pulmonary infarction in the early stages, but the combination of a normal X-ray and a normal lung scan is strong evidence that embolism and infarction have not occurred.

Pulmonary angiography is rarely indicated in the investigation of pulmonary infarction but shows characteristic abnormalities, usually much more extensive than those suggested by the plain X-ray.

Investigations

Blood. A polymorphonucleur leucocytosis often accompanies pulmonary infarction even in the absence of infection.

Serum enzymes are of little use in diagnosis since although elevation of lactic dehydrogenase and its isoenzymes is common in infarction similar changes occur in pneumonia.

ECG is of little value in diagnosis.

Arterial blood gas analysis usually shows type I respiratory failure.

Lower limb phlebography. It is important to bear in mind that pulmonary emboli may arise from any site. However, a good-quality bilateral ascending phlebogram which is completely clear of thrombus should cast doubt on the diagnosis of pulmonary thromboembolic disease and, depending upon the circumstances, may allow anticoagulant treatment to be withheld. Unfortunately, phlebography cannot be performed on all patients suspected of having pulmonary infarction but should certainly be included in the investigation of recurrent disease and, of course, when some form of surgical venous interruption or thrombectomy is being contemplated.

^{125}I *scanning of deep veins of lower limbs.* This procedure is of undoubted value in the screening of patients thought likely to develop deep venous thrombosis, but is of little use in the investigation of patients with pulmonary infarction and established venous thrombosis.

Differential diagnosis

Pulmonary infarction frequently simulates pneumonia and it is often difficult to be certain of the diagnosis. Treatment for both conditions has to be given in some cases.

Haemoptysis and pleuritic pain may suggest diagnoses of tuberculosis, bronchial carcinoma, lung abscess and bronchiectasis.

Radiologically pulmonary infarction may be mistaken for pneumonia and bronchial carcinoma.

Treatment

Considerable controversy exists about the treatment of pulmonary infarction, particularly as far as immobilization and duration of anti-coagulant therapy are concerned.

Immobilization

If phlebography has been performed and no thrombus has been outlined the patient does not need to be confined to bed. In the vast majority of patients phlebography will not have been performed and hence it is logical to assume that there may be significant thrombus remaining in the venous system and complete bed rest for a few days should be enforced in order to allow any thrombus to become more adherent to the vein wall, providing anticoagulant therapy is being given.

Anticoagulant therapy

Heparin is best given to all patients by continuous intravenous infusion for an initial period of at least two days, and preferably 5–10 days. After a loading dose of 10 000 units the rate of heparin infusion will depend upon serial laboratory coagulation tests. Oral anticoagulation with warfarin should be substituted for heparin in all cases unless an absolute contraindication exists. A period of three days overlap of heparin and warfarin treatment should be routine practice.

DURATION OF ORAL ANTICOAGULANT THERAPY

It is not logical to treat all patients for a standard period. Short-term therapy, e.g. 3–6 weeks, can be given to those patients in whom a pre-disposition to the thromboembolic event has been determined — e.g. immobilization, trauma, pregnancy, the contraceptive pill — providing the predisposing factor is no longer active. Longer duration of treatment, 3–6 months, should be considered in patients in whom the thromboembolic episode is thought to be spontaneous. Lifelong treatment should be considered in patients who develop recurrence of thromboembolism after withdrawal of anticoagulant treatment. When appropriate these patients should also be fully assessed by venography in case it is possible to perform some type of venous surgery in an attempt to prevent further embolization from the deep veins of the lower part of the body to the lungs.

Venous interruption

Venous interruption (such as caval plication or filter, or superficial femoral ligation) has a definite but very occasional place. The main indications are recurrent embolism despite well-controlled anticoagulation, and embolism or serious phlebographically proved thrombus in a patient in whom anticoagulation is contraindicated.

Prognosis

The prognosis in the majority of patients is good, providing adequate treatment is given at an early stage. Very few patients develop massive pulmonary embolism after anticoagulant therapy has been established, and only a few patients have recurrence of pulmonary infarction after the withdrawal of treatment. A high proportion of patients who develop recurrent pulmonary infarction are found to have an underlying malignant disease. Recovery from pulmonary infarction in the majority of patients is complete.

THROMBOEMBOLIC PULMONARY HYPERTENSION

Pulmonary hypertension due to recurrent pulmonary embolism is uncommon, but is usually irreversible and will ultimately prove fatal once clinical evidence of pulmonary hypertension has developed.

Fundamental points of diagnosis

Some, but by no means all, patients have a previous history of thromboembolic disease. Breathlessness on exertion associated with lightheadedness or syncope are the typical features of pulmonary hypertension. Central chest pain on exertion is also a fairly common symptom. The chest X-ray and ECG are abnormal.

Complications

Right ventricular failure invariably complicates thromboembolic pulmonary hypertension unless death is accelerated by an embolic episode.

Clinical findings

Symptoms and signs

Exertional breathlessness, lightheadedness and syncope frequently associated with angina are the symptoms. A history of thromboembolism, sometimes recurrent and often associated with pregnancy, is present in a proportion of patients. Ankle swelling is a feature of advanced disease when right ventricular failure has developed.

The physical signs are entirely cardiovascular unless there is an associated episode of pulmonary infarction. A right ventricular impulse may be palpable over the lower sternum and on auscultation of the heart the pulmonary component of the second sound is accentuated and splitting of the second sound is common. A fourth heart sound is often heard at the apex or left sternal edge. Tachycardia is usually present and the signs of right ventricular failure (raised jugular venous pressure, hepatomegaly and peripheral oedema) may be present.

Radiological examination

A chest X-ray usually shows no pulmonary abnormality except for paucity of peripheral vascular markings. The central pulmonary arteries are large and the main pulmonary artery is often very large. Cardiomegaly is a characteristic feature due to right ventricular enlargement.

Pulmonary angiography reveals occlusion of a major proportion of the pulmonary arterial system.

Perfusion lung scan is usually grossly abnormal since vascular occlusion is rarely symmetrical.

Investigations

ECG shows evidence of right ventricular hypertrophy with T-wave inversion over the right ventricle.

Arterial blood gas analysis reveals hypoxaemia without carbon dioxide retention (type I respiratory failure).

Pulmonary arterial pressure, usually measured prior to pulmonary angiography, confirms pulmonary hypertension which is usually gross if symptoms are present.

Differential diagnosis

The numerous causes of breathlessness, syncope and central chest pain have to be considered, but in practice the only alternative diagnosis is primary pulmonary hypertension.

Treatment

The treatment of thromboembolic pulmonary hypertension is generally unsatisfactory unless the disease is detected at a very early stage when long-term anticoagulant therapy may be beneficial. Usually, however, when symptoms are present treatment of any kind is ineffective. Long-term anticoagulant therapy is given to most patients and inferior vena caval plication, ligation or filter insertion is frequently performed. Alternative treatments with drugs to reduce platelet adhesiveness and to stimulate endogenous thrombolysis have also been used but with little effect. Treatment of right ventricular failure is necessary to reduce discomfort.

Prognosis

Prognosis is grave if the disease is diagnosed when severe pulmonary hypertension has become established. Only a few patients improve with treatment and the remainder die within five to ten years. Prevention offers the only hope of combating this grim complication of recurrent thromboembolic disease since the only alternative is heart-lung transplantation.

SUMMARY — SPECIAL POINTS OF EMPHASIS

• Pulmonary thromboembolic disease is the most common lung disease in hospital practice.

• The incidence of venous thrombosis and pulmonary embolism increases with age — the majority of fatal episodes occur in patients over the age of 50.

• Massive pulmonary embolism, pulmonary infarction and thrombo-embolic pulmonary hypertension are convenient clinical subdivisions of this disease, but this classification is for descriptive purposes only. In clinical practice symptoms and signs of all types of this disease may be present in the same patient and in others the clinical picture does not readily fit into one of these artificial subdivisions.

• Clinically obvious deep vein thrombosis is present in a minority of patients.

• Many patients with massive pulmonary embolism can in retrospect be seen to have had an episode of minor embolism.

• Massive pulmonary embolism frequently simulates myocardial infarction and indeed may cause myocardial infarction.

• Pulmonary angiography is the only investigation which can confirm absolutely the diagnosis of massive pulmonary embolism.

• External cardiac massage in unconscious patients with massive pulmonary embolism can cause haemodynamic improvement by fragmenting a centrally situated embolus.

• Embolectomy is rarely successful unless performed with the aid of cardiopulmonary bypass.

• Heparin should be given as soon as the diagnosis is made.

• Streptokinase can lyse emboli and improve the clinical picture rapidly.

• Pulmonary infarction often simulates other respiratory diseases, particularly pneumonia.

• Pleuritic pain and haemoptysis in any patient should always suggest a diagnosis of pulmonary infarction.

• Low-grade pyrexia, leucocytosis and non-specific radiographic pulmonary shadowing often suggest a diagnosis of infection in patients with pulmonary infarction.

• The radiographic abnormalities in pulmonary infarction are frequently bilateral and usually in the lower zones.

• In some patients it may be impossible to differentiate between pulmonary infarction and pneumonia and, therefore, treatment of both conditions has to be given.

• Thromboembolic pulmonary hypertension is a very serious complication of recurrent embolism.

• When symptoms of exertional breathlessness and syncope are present in patients with thromboembolic pulmonary hypertension treatment is usually ineffective.

• It is sometimes difficult to differentiate between thromboembolic pulmonary hypertension and primary pulmonary hypertension.

Chapter 16
Tuberculosis

INTRODUCTION

In developed countries the prevalence of tuberculosis has declined rapidly in the last few decades because of vaccination programmes, X-ray screening, improved environmental conditions and, most important of all, effective therapy. However, in some developing countries tuberculosis remains a major cause of death and morbidity and in some communities one in every hundred of the population has infectious pulmonary disease. In Britain a high proportion of patients with active disease belong to the immigrant population.

Tuberculosis is caused by infection with *Mycobacterium tuberculosis*, and although infection can occur in any organ or tissue of the body pulmonary disease is by far the most common and the most important form of tuberculosis since it provides the major source of infection. Bovine tuberculosis, and consequent infection of man with infected milk, is now virtually irradicated as a major source of disease in most Western countries.

The first infection with the tubercle bacillus results in 'primary tuberculosis', and in the vast majority of patients this occurs in the lungs. This infection is characterized by involvement of the lymph glands draining the area in which the primary focus is situated. The combination of the initial focus of infection and lymph gland involvement is called the 'primary complex'. The tonsil and cervical glands may make up the 'primary complex' in some patients with bovine tuberculosis.

Consequences of primary infection

1 In the majority of cases the infection is arrested. Later the lesions may become calcified. However, viable tubercle bacilli may remain within these 'healed' lesions for very many years.
2 Progression of the pulmonary lesion may take place and produce tuberculous pneumonia. This is uncommon.
3 Blood-borne spread of tubercle bacilli may cause acute disseminated disease, for example miliary tuberculosis and meningitis.
4 Blood-borne dissemination of organisms may occur without the production of acute disease. Tubercle bacilli, spread at the time of

primary disease, may years later cause disease in any organ, including the lung.

In young Caucasian people miliary tuberculosis, tuberculous meningitis and pleural effusion usually become manifest within a year of the primary infection, but in the elderly and non-white races the disease has no specific timetable.

The type and severity of tuberculous disease in an individual patient is dependent upon a number of important factors, including the size of the infecting dose, the virulence of the organisms and the defences of the host. Host defences may be genetically low in some races and can be reduced in others by diseases such as diabetes mellitus or by treatment with corticosteroids. Patients who have had surgical treatment for peptic ulceration and also those with pneumoconiosis, particularly silicosis, have a greater chance of developing the disease than the general population. Host defences can be increased by BCG vaccination (acquired immunity) or by the development of natural resistance.

Coincident with the development of a primary infection hypersensitivity to tuberculoprotein (a constituent of the tubercle bacillus) usually develops. This can be demonstrated by tuberculin skin testing — a positive response indicating a normal reaction to acute infection, a previous infection or BCG vaccination. The tuberculin test becomes positive within six weeks of a primary infection. After tuberculoprotein hypersensitivity has developed the tissues of the body react to tubercle bacilli in such a way that reinfection becomes very difficult. A negative response to tuberculin testing does not exclude active tuberculosis as hypersensitivity to tuberculoprotein may not develop in patients with fulminating disease.

PRIMARY PULMONARY TUBERCULOSIS

General considerations

Primary tuberculosis is most often encountered in young people, usually children, but as tuberculosis becomes less common in a community the disease may be seen in adults, especially in countries where widespread BCG vaccination is not practised.

Fundamental points of diagnosis

Diagnosis of primary pulmonary tuberculosis may be difficult, since it frequently produces little constitutional upset and it has no specific symptoms. Any symptoms in a child who has been in contact with a patient with infectious disease should be suspected as being indicative of a primary tuberculous infection. The chest X-ray may be helpful in diagnosis, but a normal X-ray does not exclude the disease. A positive tuberculin test in a child is of great diagnostic significance, much more so than in an adult.

Complications

Complications are relatively unusual and can be discussed under three headings:

1 *Extension of disease.* Local extension of disease in the lungs and general dissemination have already been discussed. Local extension occurs most often in adolescents and young adults.

2 *Mechanical complications.* Enlarged hilar lymph glands may compress the bronchi and trachea and/or caseous material may be discharged into the tracheobronchial system.

Bronchial compression can give rise to collapse of lobes or segments. For anatomical reasons the middle lobe is particularly vulnerable. Obstructive emphysema can be produced when a bronchus is almost occluded, but still allows air to pass the obstruction on inspiration. Bronchial stenosis and bronchiectasis may be the end result of pulmonary collapse caused by primary tuberculosis. Complications due to lymph node enlargement are most common in young children and adult Asians and Africans.

3 *Tuberculin hypersensitivity reactions.* Within six weeks of the primary infection hypersensitivity to tuberculoprotein develops and the tuberculin test becomes positive. This may also be accompanied by the development of erythema nodosum and phlyctenular conjunctivitis. Neither of these are, however, specifically associated with tuberculosis, since they occur in many conditions, including sarcoidosis. Phlyctenular conjunctivitis, unlike erythema nodosum, can be a manifestation of tuberculin hypersensitivity in post-primary forms of tuberculosis.

Clinical findings

Symptoms and signs

In the majority of cases the disease goes unrecognized and is either symptomless or causes mild constitutional upset, often labelled as a 'flu-like' illness. Cough occurs in patients who develop bronchial compression from enlarged hilar lymph glands when 'wheeze' may be unilateral. Distressing respiratory symptoms usually indicate rupture of a gland into a bronchus with the development of 'caseous pneumonia', extension of the primary infection, or compression of the trachea or main bronchi.

Physical signs in the chest are usually absent, but there may be a fixed rhonchus, evidence of pulmonary collapse or rarely signs of obstructive emphysema. Erythema nodosum and/or phlyctenular conjunctivitis may be the only abnormalities.

Radiological examination

In young children, especially if the X-ray has been taken when the child has been crying, interpretation is often difficult. The typical combination of a pulmonary focus and hilar glandular enlargement may be seen, but often one or other component of the 'primary complex' may not be visible. In the very young and in adult Asians and Negroes hilar glandular enlargement may be massive, but in older children and adolescents the glandular component tends to be less evident. Pulmonary lesions in the apical segment of the lower lobe may give the impression on the straight X-ray of hilar enlargement because of superimposition of shadows, and a lateral X-ray is necessary to show the true site of the lesion. Paratracheal glandular enlargement may be visible in some cases. If bronchial compression or rupture of caseous material into a bronchus has occurred there is often evidence of segmental shadowing or true pulmonary collapse. In the past these segmental pulmonary opacities caused by the mechanical effects of enlarged hilar glands were called 'epituberculosis', but this term serves no useful purpose. Occasionally there may be radiological evidence of bilateral main bronchial compression. Obstructive emphysema is rare, but is easily overlooked.

Tuberculin tests

There are three commonly used tuberculin tests:

1 Mantoux test.
2 Heaf test.
3 Tine test.

Mantoux test. Using a calibrated 1 ml tuberculin syringe and an intradermal needle 0·1 ml of a tuberculin solution (1:10 000, 1:1000 or 1:100) is injected intradermally into the volar surface of the forearm.

This intradermal injection should raise a weal and if one is not visible it means the injection has been given subcutaneously, invalidating the test.

Results are recorded after 2–3 days and expressed as the widest diameter in millimetres of induration, erythema without induration being ignored. The test is considered to be positive when there is 5 mm or more of induration. However, a 5 mm reaction to 1:100 tuberculin is unlikely to be of much clinical relevance. The most widely used tuberculin solution is 1:1000, 0·1 ml of which contains 10 TU (tuberculin units)

Heaf test. Tuberculin purified protein derivative (PPD), 100 000 units per ml, is used for this test and introduced into the skin using a Heaf multiple puncture apparatus (Heaf gun). Sterilization is performed before each test by dipping the end piece into methylated spirits and then flaming it. A drop of tuberculin is spread over about 1 cm of healthy skin (usually on the forearm away from obvious superficial veins) which is held taut by the thumb and index finger of the operator's free hand. The end plate of the Heaf gun is placed firmly on this area of skin and the handle is pressed to release the needles. Skin penetration can be pre-set to 1 mm for children and 2 mm for adults.

Tests should be read between three and seven days and the result recorded as follows:

Negative   No induration.

Grade I   Discrete palpable induration at three or more puncture sites.

Grade II   Indurated points coalesced thus producing an elevated ring.

Grade III   Induration extended to fill the central area, thus producing a coin-like lesion approximately 10 mm in diameter.

Grade IV   More extensive induration. Vesicles may form, particularly at puncture sites and there may be central sloughing of the skin.

Grades III and IV are certainly of clinical relevance but grades I and II are of doubtful significance and could possibly be associated with non-tuberculous mycobacterial infection.

Tine test. The tine unit is disposable and consists of four prongs (tines) coated with tuberculin. The tines are pressed firmly into the skin of the forearm for 2–5 seconds.

The results of tine tests read at three days can be graded in a way similar to that used for the Heaf test:

Grade I   One or two faint papules.
Grade II   Four discrete papules.
Grade III   The area encircled by the papules is completely indurated.
Grade IV   Any reaction which is greater than III, including central necrosis.

Using this grading system reactions in grades III and IV almost certainly indicate infection (current or previous) with mammalian tubercle bacilli. A grade I reaction may indicate infection with atypical mycobacteria. The significance of grade II is uncertain.

The reliability of the tine test has been questioned. False-negative results have been reported and these have probably been due to variation in the quality of units manufactured so that differing amounts of tuberculin reach the tips and outer walls of the tines and consequently the skin.

Investigations

By far the most important investigation is the *tuberculin skin test*. A strongly positive tuberculin test in a child should always be interpreted as indicating active tuberculous infection, unless it was known to be positive previously. Observed conversion of the tuberculin reaction from negative to positive in the absence of BCG vaccination provides absolute confirmation of primary infection.

It is uncommon to be able to confirm the diagnosis bacteriologically. Attempts should be made by examination of sputum (when present), laryngeal swabs, gastric washings or from trap specimens or biopsies and washings at bronchoscopy. In all cases vigorous attempts must be made to trace the source of infection in order to ascertain the drug sensitivity pattern of the infecting organism.

Bronchoscopy may be necessary in patients with evidence of major pulmonary collapse, bilateral main bronchus compression or when glandular enlargement is suspected of compressing or eroding the trachea. In patients with obstructive emphysema bronchoscopy is also indicated in order to attempt to restore a bronchial lumen whenever possible by removal of caseous material, and also to exclude other causes of obstructive emphysema such as foreign body inhalation.

Differential diagnosis

There are few conditions which can be mistaken for primary pulmonary tuberculosis when the chest X-ray is abnormal, the tuberculin test is positive and there is a history of contact with the disease. However, simple pneumonia and foreign body inhalation have always to be considered in children, and in older patients other causes of hilar glandular enlargement such as sarcoidosis and malignant disease may have to be excluded.

Treatment

Antituberculosis drug treatment is indicated in all patients in whom a confident diagnosis of primary tuberculosis has been made. In young children under the age of five a strongly positive tuberculin test should itself be regarded as evidence of primary infection requiring treatment, providing the child has not received BCG vaccination.

Antituberculosis drug treatment

Primary tuberculosis should be treated in the same way as post-primary pulmonary tuberculosis (*see* p. 246). In most cases treatment with two drugs throughout is sufficient, particularly when the presumed source of infection indicates fully sensitive organisms.

Corticosteroid therapy

Corticosteroid therapy should be given as well as antituberculosis drug therapy to patients who have evidence of major bronchial occlusion (p. 237).

Bronchoscopy

See under Complications above.

Prognosis

Most patients with primary pulmonary tuberculosis recover spontaneously. With treatment the prognosis is excellent since all tubercle bacilli are killed and reactivation in later life is, therefore, prevented. Even with treatment, however, it may not always be possible to prevent the development of bronchostenosis and bronchiectasis if there is pulmonary collapse due to bronchial occlusion at the time of diagnosis.

MILIARY TUBERCULOSIS

General considerations

Untreated miliary tuberculosis is almost always fatal. There are two clinical varieties — acute and chronic cryptic. Acute disease can occur at all ages, but young children are particularly at risk since their resistance to haematogenous dissemination of tubercle bacilli is poor. Measles and whooping cough appear to aid the development of acute miliary tuberculosis in children, and in adults chronic diseases (e.g. leukaemia) and corticosteroid therapy can be predisposing factors. Chronic cryptic disease usually occurs in adults, especially the elderly, and this type of miliary tuberculosis is now more common than the acute form in some developed countries. Chronic miliary tuberculosis presents a difficult clinical problem and the diagnosis is not infrequently made at autopsy.

Tuberculous meningitis often accompanies miliary disease, especially in children. Miliary tuberculosis and meningitis are virtually unknown in children previously vaccinated with BCG.

Fundamental points of diagnosis

ACUTE MILIARY TUBERCULOSIS

The classical features of this form of the disease are an acute or subacute febrile illness, the presence of choroidal tubercles, and uniform miliary shadowing throughout both lung fields on the chest X-ray.

CHRONIC CRYPTIC MILIARY TUBERCULOSIS

Diagnosis is difficult and it is often overlooked because of a lack of appreciation of its insidious nature and the numerous ways in which it can present. Weight loss, malaise, low-grade pyrexia and a number of haematological disorders (*see below*) may be manifestations of this disease. The chest X-ray may be abnormal, but the absence of classical miliary mottling does not exclude the diagnosis.

The tuberculin test in miliary tuberculosis

The tuberculin test in most cases of miliary tuberculosis is strongly positive. However, in a few cases of overwhelming acute disease it can be negative, and in a higher proportion of patients with chronic disease it may also be misleadingly negative. Nevertheless, it must be emphasized that the tuberculin test is an important investigation since it is strongly positive in the majority of patients.

Complications

Acute miliary tuberculosis is often accompanied by tuberculous meningitis. Tuberculous pleural effusion may also develop but the majority of cases of tuberculous pleural effusion are seen without evidence of miliary disease.

Chronic cryptic disease may produce a number of blood dyscrasias including pancytopenia, 'leukaemoid reaction', aplastic anaemia, agranulocytosis, leucoerythroblastic anaemia and polycythaemia.

Hypokalaemia can occur in all forms of miliary tuberculosis but is most common in middle-aged and elderly patients.

Hyponatraemia due to inappropriate ADH secretion is a well-recognized feature of extensive tuberculosis of any type.

Clinical features

Symptoms and signs

ACUTE MILIARY DISEASE

There are no specific symptoms of miliary tuberculosis. The onset of the disease may be gradual or sudden and symptoms are those of any febrile illness unless tuberculous meningitis also develops. Respiratory symptoms are uncommon, but cough and breathlessness may develop in advanced cases.

There are usually no abnormal clinical findings on examination of the lungs. A few fine crepitations may be audible in patients with extensive pulmonary involvement. The most important physical finding is the recognition of choroidal tubercles. Efficient use of the ophthalmoscope may be very difficult in the irritable child, even after the pupils have been dilated, and in some cases it may be necessary to give sedation or even an anaesthetic to allow adequate visualization of the fundi. Choroidal tubercles are usually less than one quarter of the diameter of the optic disc, and initially are yellow, shiny and slightly raised. Older tubercles are white and flat. They may be scanty or numerous, but the recognition of one characteristic tubercle is diagnostic.

Splenomegaly occurs in approximately 50% of patients with acute miliary disease, and there may also be hepatomegaly.

CHRONIC CRYPTIC DISEASE

The symptoms of chronic disease are protean, and chronic ill health of any description can be produced by this condition.

Choroidal tubercles are rarely seen, but a thorough search should always be made. Pyrexia is usually a feature but is often low-grade. Hepatosplenomegaly occurs in some patients and there may be enlargement of cervical lymph glands.

Progressive ill-health associated with weight loss, pyrexia and a haematological abnormality is the most common picture in elderly patients.

Radiological examination

A normal chest X-ray does not exclude a diagnosis of miliary tuberculosis. When miliary lesions (round shadows 1·5–3 mm in diameter) are visible they are usually evenly distributed throughout the lung fields, but in early cases are often best seen in the peripheral areas of the intercostal spaces. Larger pulmonary shadows (up to 10 mm in diameter) are seen in some patients and there may be evidence of the primary tuberculous complex or post-primary disease. Occasionally there are pleural effusions which may be bilateral.

Investigations

The *tuberculin test* is an important investigation which must be performed in all cases even though it may be misleadingly negative in a small number of patients (*see above*). A strongly positive tuberculin reaction in the young or the elderly is always of great diagnostic importance.

Bacteriological confirmation of disease is often difficult but should be attempted by examination of sputum, laryngeal swabs, gastric lavage and early morning urine specimens. Direct examination of bone marrow for tubercle bacilli and tubercles may give an immediate diagnosis, and specimens of bone marrow should always be cultured for tubercle bacilli. In patients with meningitis bacteriological confirmation may be obtained from direct examination or culture of CSF. It is vital to have all specimens thoroughly examined directly by an expert since rarely is it possible to delay a decision about institution of treatment until the results of cultures are available.

Histological examination of liver biopsy specimens may establish the diagnosis, and whenever possible the liver biopsy should also be cultured.

THERAPEUTIC TRIAL OF ANTITUBERCULOSIS DRUGS

In a number of patients, especially with the chronic cryptic form of the disease, confirmation of the disease is impossible and a trial of treatment has to be used diagnostically. Whenever it is decided to institute a therapeutic trial of antituberculosis drugs it is important that combinations of isoniazid, ethambutol and PAS (usually isoniazid and ethambutol) should be used since these drugs are specifically active against tubercle bacilli. Combinations of drugs including rifampicin and streptomycin may give misleading results because of their potent antibacterial properties. If pyrexia is abolished within two weeks of a therapeutic trial of specific antituberculosis drugs this is virtually diagnostic and the drug combination may then be modified if necessary.

Differential diagnosis

In the absence of choroidal tubercles and miliary shadowing on X-ray the differential diagnosis includes all causes of pyrexia and general ill-health.

Sarcoidosis may cause pulmonary lesions which radiologically appear similar to those of miliary tuberculosis, but patients with sarcoidosis are usually symptomless and very rarely have pyrexia. Coalworker's pneumoconiosis, silicosis and multiple haematogenous metastatic malignant lesions can also produce X-ray changes which may be confused with miliary tuberculosis.

Treatment

Antituberculosis drug therapy is the same as for post-primary pulmonary tuberculosis (*see* p. 252)

Corticosteroid therapy should be given to all patients who are desperately ill and who have tuberculous meningitis.

Prognosis

Providing antituberculosis treatment is given, together with corticosteroid therapy when indicated, the prognosis of this once almost invariably fatal disease is good. Patients with miliary tuberculosis not associated with tuberculous meningitis usually recover completely. In some patients with tuberculous meningitis, however, neurological sequelae cannot be prevented.

POST-PRIMARY PULMONARY TUBERCULOSIS

General considerations

Post-primary pulmonary tuberculosis (pulmonary tuberculosis) most often develops because of reactivation of a quiescent primary infection. Direct progression of the primary infection is less common but can occur especially in young adults and in African and Asian children. Exogenous superinfection directly causing pulmonary tuberculosis is uncommon.

Pulmonary tuberculosis is the most important form of disease since it is the major source of infection. However, because a quiescent primary lesion may break down years later successful treatment of all cases of infectious pulmonary tuberculosis would only result in a total eradication of the disease when those members of the community with untreated primary and non-infectious lesions had died from other causes or had been treated with antituberculosis drugs. Contact-tracing in pulmonary tuberculosis is mainly to detect cases of primary disease caused by the index case and not to find a source of infection, except in the relatively rare event of pulmonary tuberculosis developing by progression of a primary infection.

Fundamental points of diagnosis

The possibility of tuberculosis must be borne in mind in any pulmonary disease irrespective of the clinical features and radiological findings. In typical cases the X-ray features are strongly suggestive of the diagnosis but examination of sputum for tubercle bacilli must not be confined to patients with classical disease. It is a wise precaution to have sputum examined for tubercle bacilli in all patients with a chest X-ray abnormality if a definitive alternative diagnosis has not been made, and even then it must be remembered that tuberculosis can complicate diseases such as silicosis, or be activated by corticosteroid therapy for other conditions.

Complications

PULMONARY DESTRUCTION

The major complication of pulmonary tuberculosis is irreversible pulmonary destruction. Although treatment can now be expected to eradicate the infection in all cases, an early death from cor pulmonale and respiratory failure cannot be prevented in patients who had previously sustained extensive lung damage. Even mild disease will leave 'post-tuberculous bronchiectasis' but fortunately, since tuberculosis most commonly involves the upper lobes, this form of bronchiectasis rarely produces symptoms because it is efficiently drained by gravity.

PLEURAL COMPLICATIONS

Tuberculous pleurisy is a relatively frequent complication of pulmonary tuberculosis and pleural effusion may develop in acute cases. Tuberculous empyema is now uncommon in developed countries but still occurs after rupture of a tuberculous cavity into the pleural space leading to pyopneumothorax.

TUBERCULOUS LARYNGITIS

This is usually a complication of extensive pulmonary disease with positive sputum.

DISSEMINATED TUBERCULOSIS

Pulmonary tuberculosis may be the source of dissemination to other organs in patients in whom the disease has developed by extension of the primary infection, or in whom the disease has been induced by corticosteroid therapy.

INTRACAVITARY ASPERGILLOMA

Fungal colonizaton, usually with *Aspergillus fumigatus,* of cavities remaining in the lung after treatment is common (*see* p. 125). Fungal colonization of active disease is rare.

HYPOKALAEMIA

Hypokalaemia may complicate severe acute disease.

HYPONATRAEMIA

Hyponatraemia, often associated with inappropriate ADH production, is found in some patients with extensive disease.

AMYLOIDOSIS

Amyloidosis is a complication of chronic pulmonary tuberculosis and tuberculous empyema which are now uncommon in developed countries.

CARCINOMA OF BRONCHUS

A definite association of tuberculosis and bronchial carcinoma has not been proved but it is not uncommon for bronchial carcinoma to develop in areas of healed tuberculosis—'scar tumours'.

Clinical findings

Symptoms and signs

There are no specific symptoms of pulmonary tuberculosis; many patients with quite extensive disease diagnosed by X-ray screening may deny symptoms.

The symptoms are lassitude, weight loss, night sweats, cough productive of mucoid sputum, and haemoptysis. Constitutional symptoms are prominent in acute disease, whereas respiratory symptoms without much constitutional upset are common in chronic disease. Distressing respiratory symptoms usually indicate extensive disease. Breathlessness, in the absence of pleural effusion or pyopneumothorax, only occurs when extensive pulmonary destruction or consolidation has developed. Sputum is usually scanty and mucoid. Copious purulent sputum is evidence of gross pulmonary damage with superadded bacterial infection. Haemoptysis may be recurrent, massive and occasionally fatal.

Night sweats certainly occur in acute disease, but not all patients with tuberculosis sweat excessively at night, and by no means all patients with sleep sweats have tuberculosis.

The physical findings in pulmonary tuberculosis are also in no way specific. Frequently, there may be no abnormalities on clinical examination even though extensive disease may be shown on X-ray. This disparity between the physical and X-ray findings is helpful diagnostically, since it is rarely encountered in bacterial pneumonia, but it can be a feature of other diseases such as sarcoidosis. The classical findings in pulmonary tuberculosis are upper zone crepitations, but there may be evidence of consolidation, bronchiectasis and gross pulmonary fibrosis. Bronchial breath sounds in tuberculosis usually indicate consolidation, a shrunken and fibrotic lobe supplied by a patent bronchus, or a large pulmonary cavity. Fever is present in most patients with acute and subacute disease, but may be absent in patients with extensive chronic disease. Finger clubbing is not a feature of tuberculosis unless there is gross pulmonary destruction with superadded bacterial infection, or tuberculous empyema.

Radiological examination

Radiological examination of the chest is much more informative than clinical examination and is the most important examination in the diagnosis of pulmonary tuberculosis. A normal chest X-ray virtually excludes pulmonary tuberculosis, although it is possible for the very rare endobronchial tuberculosis or tuberculous bronchitis to be present in the absence of a radiological abnormality.

The X-ray abnormalities which should immediately suggest a diagnosis of tuberculosis are:

Upper zone shadows (unilateral or bilateral)

Cavitated upper lobe abnormalities.

The radiological abnormalities in tuberculosis are often much more extensive than the clinical features suggest. Tuberculosis can imitate any pulmonary pathology such as pneumonia and bronchial carcinoma. The presence of calcification within a pulmonary abnormality suggests a tuberculous aetiology but is not diagnostic since simple inflammatory lesions and malignant tumours may develop in areas of lung previously damaged by a tuberculous infection. Benign tumours may also contain calcified elements.

In chronic pulmonary tuberculosis it is not uncommon to see gross shrinkage of the upper lobes with elevation of one or both hilar shadows.

Investigations

SPUTUM EXAMINATION

The diagnosis of pulmonary tuberculosis is confirmed by the finding of acid- and alcohol-fast bacilli in smears of sputum stained by the Ziehl–Neelsen method (or by the use of fluorescent microscopy techniques) or by the culture of tubercle bacilli from sputum. It must be emphasized that a specific request must be made for the bacteriologist to examine sputum for tubercle bacilli, and that a positive culture may take many weeks to be reported. The absence of tubercle bacilli in smears of sputum does not exclude a diagnosis of tuberculosis, but in most cases of extensive disease, especially if cavitated, a positive direct smear result can be anticipated.

At least three specimens of sputum should be submitted for bacteriological examination, and since patients with scanty sputum are more likely to produce adequate specimens immediately after waking early morning specimens are ideal.

It must be assumed that the results of drug sensitivity tests may not be available for up to three months since these involve subculture of a primary culture.

LARYNGEAL SWABS AND GASTRIC LAVAGE

In patients who do not produce sputum or immediately swallow it, laryngeal swabs or gastric lavage specimens taken first thing in the morning may have to be examined instead of sputum. Inability to produce sputum is particularly common in children and women. In adult patients the skills of a physiotherapist should be employed to try to obtain a specimen of sputum before resorting to gastric lavage. Laryngeal swabs and gastric lavage specimens are not usually suitable for direct smear examination.

TUBERCULIN TEST

The tuberculin test is a valuable diagnostic aid which tends to be overlooked in countries where tuberculosis is now uncommon.

HAEMATOLOGICAL INDICES

Active tuberculosis is usually accompanied by elevation, often gross, of the erythrocyte sedimentation rate, but this is not a reliable indicator of disease activity. The white cell count is usually normal or low, but in some cases there may be a mild leucocytosis.

BRONCHOSCOPY

When a chest X-ray suggests active tuberculosis and the patient has no sputum, or when it is scanty and negative on direct smear for tubercle bacilli, fibreoptic bronchoscopy can be used to obtain bronchial brushings, washings and transbronchial lung biopsy specimens. In these patients with suggestive X-rays fibreoptic bronchoscopy can provide immediate confirmation of disease in approximately 50%, and the diagnostic rate rises to about 70% when cultures become available.

Bronchoscopy is, of course, indicated in sputum-negative patients in whom the diagnosis is in doubt, mainly to exclude bronchial carcinoma. Biopsy of abnormal mucosa may yield a positive histological diagnosis in endobronchial tuberculosis.

PLEURAL BIOPSY

Pleural biopsy (p. 170) and examination of pleural liquid is necessary to establish a diagnosis of tuberculous pleural effusion.

Differential diagnosis

Tuberculosis is a great imitator and, therefore, it must be included in the diagnosis of any pulmonary disease associated with cough and sputum, especially if the X-ray is abnormal. Bronchial carcinoma and suppurative pneumonia are commonly difficult differential diagnostic problems, but rarer diseases such as sarcoidosis and pulmonary eosinophilia may also produce radiological abnormalities very similar to those of pulmonary tuberculosis.

Treatment

Antituberculosis drug treatment is indicated in all patients with active disease. Bed rest is not necessary unless the patient is too ill to be up and about. Strict isolation is not required in all cases and is never necessary for long because the patient becomes non-infectious within 2–4 weeks of being given effective treatment.

There are a number of very important principles which govern the drug treatment of tuberculosis:

1 To avoid development of drug resistance a combination of drugs (at least two) must be used. Initially, to cover the possibility of primary resistance to one drug, at least three drugs should be given until drug sensitivity patterns of the organism are known. The only exception to this rule is chemoprophylaxis (*see* p. 259).
2 Drugs must be taken regularly during the treatment period to avoid the development of acquired drug resistance.

3 Duration of treatment necessary to achieve cure depends upon the drug combination used.

4 If a patient has been previously treated with antituberculosis drugs and has relapsed it must be assumed that the organisms are resistant to the drugs used until drug sensitivity reports are available.

5 All drugs are given in single daily doses together (except PAS). When combinations including rifampicin are used the drugs should be taken one hour before breakfast.

Drug regimens

A number of different drug combinations are effective. The duration of the treatment course depends upon the combination of drugs used during the maintenance phase of therapy, i.e. after the initial phase of triple or quadruple drug treatment.

SIX MONTHS TREATMENT

The total duration of therapy need not exceed six months when a combination of isoniazid and rifampicin is preceded by a two-month phase of treatment with these drugs *plus* pyrazinamide and ethambutol or streptomycin.

NINE MONTHS TREATMENT

The total duration of therapy need not exceed nine months when a combination of isoniazid and rifampicin is used following an initial period of triple drug therapy (two months) with these drugs in combination with ethambutol or streptomycin.

LONGER DURATION TREATMENT

Because other drugs are less effective, therapy with drug combinations other than isoniazid and rifampicin should be given for 18 months. In some cases of minimal disease a total duration of 12 months may be sufficient.

Choice of drug combination

In patients in whom primary drug resistance is not suspected a drug combination of isoniazid, rifampicin plus ethambutol or streptomycin should be chosen for the initial phase of treatment lasting two months. Thereafter, providing the organisms are sensitive, treatment with isoniazid and rifampicin should be continued to complete a total treatment course of nine months. Alternatively the shorter course treatment lasting six months using an initial four-drug combination of isoniazid, rifampicin, pyrazinamide and ethambutol or streptomycin for two months can be chosen. Compliance is almost certainly improved by short-course therapy and the six and nine months regimens can be considered to be the treatments of choice. However, drug toxicity, drug resistance, and in some underdeveloped countries the cost of treatment, especially with rifampicin, may make it necessary to use other drug combinations. Alternative drug combinations for the continuation phase of treatment are:

Isoniazid plus ethambutol
Isoniazid plus PAS
(Isoniazid plus thioacetazone).

The combination of isoniazid and thioacetazone is rarely used except in countries where other regimens cannot be used because of expense.

Intermittent regimens

Intermittent regimens have been developed to cut down the cost of treatment and also to overcome problems with patient compliance. A number of intermittent drug combinations have been shown to be effective. The combination of streptomycin and high-dose isoniazid given twice weekly is occasionally used in developed countries as supervised therapy for poorly compliant patients, since the isoniazid is given at the same time as the injection of streptomycin.

Antituberculosis drugs

First-line drugs:
Isoniazid
Rifampicin
Ethambutol
Streptomycin
Pyrazinamide.

Alternative drugs:
PAS (sodium aminosalicylate)
Thioacetazone.

Second-line drugs:
Capreomycin
Cycloserine
Ethionamide
Viomycin
Kanamycin.

The second-line drugs are rarely used except for treatment of patients with drug-resistant organisms, or severe hypersensitivity reactions to other drugs.

ISONIAZID

Antituberculosis activity. High.

Administration. Oral. Single daily dose (preparations for intramuscular and intrathecal administration available).

Dosage. Standard adult dose of 300 mg. Children — 3 mg/kg body weight (10 mg/kg in tuberculous meningitis). 14 mg/kg when given twice weekly with streptomycin. In chemoprophylaxis 5 mg/kg (*see* p. 260).

Side-effects. Adverse reactions to isoniazid are rare, but when hypersensitivity reactions do occur they can be severe. Fever, rash, lymphadenopathy, blood dyscrasias, encephalopathy, jaundice and renal impairment can occur.

Peripheral neuropathy is the most common side-effect. Drowsiness, inability to concentrate, vertigo, euphoria, hyper-reflexia, psychoses and epileptiform fits can be produced in susceptible individuals by high-dose treatment. Neurotoxic features, in particular peripheral neuropathy, may be prevented by concurrent treatment with pyridoxine 10–20 mg daily. Pyridoxine should be given routinely to patients receiving high-dose isoniazid treatment (above 10 mg/kg).

RIFAMPICIN

Antituberculosis activity. High.

Administration. Oral or intravenous. Once daily one hour before breakfast (absorption impaired if given orally with food).

Dosage. Standard adult doses of 600 mg for patients above 50 kg and 450 mg if below 50 kg. Children — 20 mg/kg with a maximum daily dose of 600 mg.

Side-effects. The urine becomes orange-red in colour and all patients should be informed of this expected occurrence. A similar colour change of sputum, sweat and tears may be noticed.

Toxic effects are uncommon during continuous treatment. Hypersensitivity reactions are rare. The most common adverse reactions involve liver function. Transient elevations of serum transaminases and bilirubin are relatively common in the early weeks of treatment and do not necessarily indicate withdrawal of therapy, unless the blood abnormalities are progressive.

Jaundice may be induced by hypersensitivity, sometimes in combination with isoniazid hypersensitivity, but also by metabolic competition for excretion pathways of bilirubin in the liver.

Very uncommon toxic effects include leucopenia, thrombocytopenia and haematolytic anaemia. Pancreatitis and renal impairment have also been described.

If rifampicin is given intermittently side-effects are much more common and include skin flushing and itching, abdominal pain, nausea and diarrhoea, a 'flu' syndrome, breathlessness and wheeze, purpura and acute renal failure.

Enzyme induction. Rifampicin induces metabolizing enzymes in the liver, which can cause problems with:
  Anticoagulant therapy
  Corticosteroid therapy
  Digoxin therapy
  Treatment of diabetes with oral drugs
  Oral contraception.

Pregnancy. Patients using oral contraception must be warned of the increased liability to become pregnant while receiving rifampicin. Alternative methods of contraception should be advised. Although no cases of human teratogenicity have been reported rifampicin should be avoided during pregnancy since teratogenic effects have been observed in animals given very high doses.

ETHAMBUTOL

Antituberculosis activity.   Moderate.

Administration.   Oral, single daily dose.

Dosage.   15 mg/kg body weight. 25 mg/kg in the initial period of treatment, for short-course regimen and if a combination of only two drugs including ethambutol has been chosen.

Side-effects.   Hypersensitivity reactions are uncommon. The most important toxic effect is retrobulbar neuritis, which usually presents with reduced visual acuity, contraction of the visual fields and colour vision changes. All patients taking ethambutol should be specifically advised to seek medical attention should they develop any visual problems. However, visual toxicity is rare with a dose of 15 mg/kg, but may occur in patients with impaired renal function. Regular checks of visual function are not required in patients with normal kidneys, but ethambutol is best avoided in children because of the difficulty of early symptomatic detection of visual disturbances. In the majority of cases the visual abnormalities are reversible after withdrawal of treatment but recovery may take up to a year.

Pregnancy.   Ethambutol is best avoided during pregnancy, but no cases of human teratogenicity have been reported.

STREPTOMYCIN

Antituberculosis activity.   High.

Administration.   Intramuscular injection once daily (special preparations are available for intrathecal use).

Dosage.   The standard adult doses are 1 g for patients under the age of 40 and 0·75 g for patients over the age of 40.
    Streptomycin treatment should be monitored by blood levels. The serum level of streptomycin, 24 hours after the last injection, should not exceed 2 μg/ml.

Side-effects.   Hypersensitivity reactions with rash, fever and haematological abnormalities are not uncommon.

The most important toxic effect is vestibular disturbance which presents with dizziness and unsteady gait. Deafness is uncommon and is usually confined to high sound frequencies. As with other aminoglycosides proximal renal tubular damage may occur. Streptomycin is best avoided in patients with renal disease.

Rare side-effects include: nausea, headache, flushing, tingling round the mouth, potentiation of neuromuscular blocking drugs, blood dyscrasias, and congenital deafness when given during pregnancy.

PYRAZINAMIDE

Antituberculosis activity.   High.

Administration.   Oral single daily dose.

Dosage.   1·5 g for patients less than 50 kg, 2·0 g for patients who weigh between 50 and 75 kg and 2·5 g for patients with a body weight of over 75 kg.

Side-effects.   The most important is hepatitis which is usually preceded by nausea and vomiting. Hypersensitivity reactions, arthralgia and skin photosensitivity may occur.

Pyrazinamide readily crosses the blood–brain barrier and should be used in the treatment of tuberculous meningitis.

PAS (SODIUM AMINOSALICYLATE)

Antituberculosis activity.   Weak.

Administration.   Oral in divided daily doses.

Dosage.   The total daily dose is 10–20 g (300 mg/kg). A daily dose of 15 g is usually chosen. Single daily dosage treatment is not usually possible because of gastrointestinal side-effects. Individual divided doses must not be less than 5 g.

Side-effects.   Gastrointestinal problems are particularly common and these include nausea, vomiting and diarrhoea. Also, PAS occasionally causes malabsorption and hence should be avoided in patients who have had gastric surgery. Hypersensitivity reactions are more common than with other antituberculosis drugs. Other toxic effects are anaemia, goitre, prolongation of the prothrombin time and hypokalaemia. The high sodium content of most preparations of PAS may precipitate cardiac failure.

Because of its toxicity and low antituberculosis activity PAS is rarely used in countries where the expense of the newer, less toxic and more effective drugs does not prevent their use. Children appear to tolerate PAS better than adults.

THIOACETAZONE

Antituberculosis activity.   Weak.

Administration.   Oral (single daily doses in most regimens).

Dosage.   2 mg/kg body weight.

Side-effects.   Numerous minor side-effects such as nausea, vomiting, flushing, itchiness of the skin and dizziness may occur in the early weeks of treatment.

The most serious toxic effects are haemolytic anaemia, thrombocytopenia, agranulocytosis, erythema multiforme, cerebral oedema, and liver dysfunction.

Toxic reactions to thioacetazone are more common in certain races, e.g. Chinese. Thioacetazone is mainly used as a cheap companion drug to isoniazid in underdeveloped countries.

Hypersensitivity reactions

The most common manifestations of drug hypersensitivity are fever and rash. Unless the patient is desperately ill, when corticosteroid therapy may have to be used to suppress drug hypersensitivity, all drugs should be discontinued until the reaction has subsided. Provocative doses of the individual drugs should then be given on separate days. Full doses can be used if the reaction is mild, but with moderate or severe reactions the provocative dose should be small or minute. The production of the signs of hypersensitivity will indicate the drug or drugs to which the patient has developed hypersensitivity. In the case of single-drug hypersensitivity treatment can be restarted with the drug or drugs shown not to induce a reaction, in combination, if necessary, with another antituberculosis drug. When multiple drug hypersensitivity is demonstrated desensitization to drugs may have to be attempted, or corticosteroid cover given to suppress hypersensitivity reactions.

Corticosteroid therapy

Corticosteroid therapy *plus* antituberculosis drug treatment is indicated:

1 In moribund patients in an attempt to keep them alive, perhaps by suppressing tuberculoprotein hypersensitivity, until antituberculosis treatment has had time to take effect.
2 In tuberculous meningitis, in an attempt to prevent fibrosis and subsequent neurological sequelae.
3 In tuberculous pleural effusions to prevent pleural fibrosis and to promote resorption of fluid to avoid repeated pleural aspirations.
4 In tuberculous pericarditis, peritonitis and genitourinary disease to prevent fibrosis giving rise to adhesions and strictures.
5 In primary pulmonary tuberculosis if mediastinal glandular enlargement has produced bronchial obstruction.
6 To suppress drug hypersensitivity reactions when treatment cannot be discontinued or attempts at desensitization have failed.
7 In adrenal disease as replacement therapy.

In the majority of cases it is sufficient to give prednisolone in a daily dose of 20–40 mg for a period of six weeks and then to withdraw treatment over a period of a few weeks. In children the dose should be calculated according to body weight: 2 mg/kg for children under the age of two, 1·5 mg/kg in those aged two to ten, and 1 mg/kg for older children. Replacement therapy is usually by hydrocortisone with or without the addition of fludrocortisone and is life-long.

Chemoprophylaxis (isoniazid 5 mg/kg body weight)

Primary chemoprophylaxis means the treatment of uninfected tuberculin-negative individuals to prevent development of disease. This is usually unnecessary except in the case of some breast-fed infants who cannot be separated from a mother with tuberculosis. Isoniazid-resistant BCG may be given simultaneously.

Secondary chemoprophylaxis means the treatment of infected tuberculin-positive individuals to prevent clinical disease. This is sometimes given to:

1   Children under the age of five with strongly positive tuberculin reactions.

2   Older children who because of recent contact with the disease are believed to have had recent tuberculin conversion from negative to positive.

3   Known recent tuberculin converters of any age.

4   Patients with evidence of previous untreated pulmonary disease (e.g. calcified pulmonary lesions) who require long-term corticosteroid therapy for other diseases such as bronchial asthma or temporal arteritis.

Isoniazid in a single daily dose of 5 mg/kg is used without a companion drug for chemoprophylaxis in some countries. Many physicians, however, prefer to use conventional two-drug chemotherapy for the indications listed under secondary chemoprophylaxis.

SUMMARY — SPECIAL POINTS OF EMPHASIS

• A positive tuberculin test indicates active infection, a previous infection or BCG vaccination.

• Any suggestive symptom in a child under the age of five who has had contact with infectious disease should be regarded as indicative of tuberculous infection.

• Conversion of the tuberculin test from negative to positive in the absence of BCG vaccination is confirmation of tuberculous infection.

• The complications of primary TB are (1) local extension and general dissemination, (2) mechanical compression of bronchi by enlarged glands, (3) the development of tuberculoprotein hypersensitivity reactions.

• Miliary tuberculosis may be acute or chronic.

• Miliary TB is almost always fatal without specific treatment.

• Visualization of choroidal tubercles is confirmation of a diagnosis of miliary TB.

• Chronic cryptic miliary TB often has no specific features and the diagnosis may have to be made by a therapeutic trial of specific antituberculosis drugs.

• Haematological abnormalities are common in chronic cryptic miliary TB.

- Pulmonary tuberculosis is a great dissembler and should be suspected in any patient with an X-ray abnormality if a secure alternative diagnosis has not been established.

- It is a wise precaution to have sputum examined for tubercle bacilli in all patients with a chest X-ray abnormality if a definitive alternative diagnosis has not been established.

- The physical findings in pulmonary TB may be few even when the X-ray shows extensive disease.

- X-ray abnormalities in the upper zones, especially if cavitated, should always raise the suspicion of pulmonary TB.

- The results of drug sensitivity tests may not be available for up to three months.

- Strict compliance is imperative and all patients must be persuaded to take treatment regularly and to report possible side-effects early.

Further reading

James D.J. & Studdy P.R. (1981) *A Colour Atlas of Respiratory Diseases.* London: Wolfe Medical Publications.
Ross J.D. & Horne N.W. (1983) *Modern Drug Treatment in Tuberculosis,* 6th Edition. London: The Chest, Heart and Stroke Association.

Chapter 17
Sarcoidosis

General considerations

Sarcoidosis is a systemic granulomatous disease of undetermined aetiology and pathogenesis. It has a worldwide distribution but may be less common in tropical than temperate areas. The highest incidence is in young adults, and females appear to develop the disease more often than males.

The hilar glands and lungs are more often involved than any other tissues of the body, but liver, spleen, skin, eyes, phalangeal bones and parotid glands are not infrequent sites. In pulmonary sarcoidosis there is a vast increase in the number of T-lymphocytes within the alveolar structures.

The Kveim reaction is positive in many patients and tuberculin-type skin hypersensitivities are frequently depressed. Many cases are asymptomatic and, therefore, go unrecognized, or the diagnosis is made by routine chest X-ray. Erythema nodosum is commonly associated with sarcoidosis, particularly when hilar glands are involved. Pulmonary sarcoidosis may coincide with hilar glandular disease or may occur without evidence of glandular involvement. Pleural sarcoidosis is extremely uncommom.

Fundamental points of diagnosis

Radiological evidence of bilateral symmetrical hilar glandular enlargement in the presence of erythema nodosum presents the typical picture which in itself is virtually diagnostic. Pulmonary sarcoidosis, not associated with hilar adenopathy, is a much more difficult problem since the radiological features are often indistinguishable from other conditions. Confirmatory histological evidence of epithelioid tubercles with little or no necrosis and/or a positive Kveim test are usually necessary in these cases.

Complications

The major pulmonary complication of sarcoidosis is progressive fibrosis which in the lung can result in gross disturbance of function leading to death from cor pulmonale and respiratory failure.

Involvement of other organs and tissues can lead to a wide variety of complications:

Eye — loss of vision.

Heart — conduction disorders, cardiac failure or sudden death.

Nervous system — fits, dysfunction of the hypothalamus and pituitary, cranial nerve lesions and peripheral neuropathies.

Alimentary system — hypersplenism.

Skeletal system — cystic osteitis and progressive disorganization of the terminal phalanges.

Skin — disfiguring skin lesions including lupus pernio.

Abnormal calcium metabolism

In some cases of chronic widespread sarcoidosis an increased sensitivity to vitamin D can lead to hypercalcaemia and hypercalciuria. Calcium deposition in the kidneys may impair renal function. Symptoms of hypercalcaemia such as lethargy and muscular weakness are uncommon.

Clinical findings

Symptoms and signs

Respiratory symptoms are uncommon unless gross pulmonary fibrosis causes breathlessness. Cough may be troublesome if there is extensive pulmonary damage, but cough can also be a feature of bronchial involvement. Infiltration of the bronchi with sarcoid tissue is rare, but occurs even in the absence of gross pulmonary involvement and should be suspected if cough is present in patients with hilar glandular enlargement.

Erythema nodosum, and arthralgia without skin lesions, are usually the only clinical manifestations of hilar glandular disease.

Clinical examination of the chest is of little value. Indeed the absence of physical signs in the presence of gross radiological abnormality is a diagnostic feature. Extensive pulmonary fibrosis may produce non-specific signs. Cervical lymph node enlargement often accompanies mediastinal lymphadenopathy. This is said to be more common in the right scalene area. Sarcoid granulomas in the nose are common in cases of intrathoracic sarcoidosis and examination of the nasal mucosa should be routine in all cases.

Radiological examination

The chest X-ray is often used to 'stage' the disease (Fig 17.1):

Stage 0   Normal chest X-ray (diagnosis having been made by biopsy of neck gland, skin, etc.).

Stage 1   Bilateral hilar adenopathy, often in conjunction with evidence of mediastinal glandular involvement particularly in the right paratracheal region.

Stage 2   Bilateral hilar adenopathy plus evidence of pulmonary infiltration.

Stage 3   Pulmonary infiltration with normal hilar shadows.

Overt evidence of irreversible damage to the lung parenchyma such as

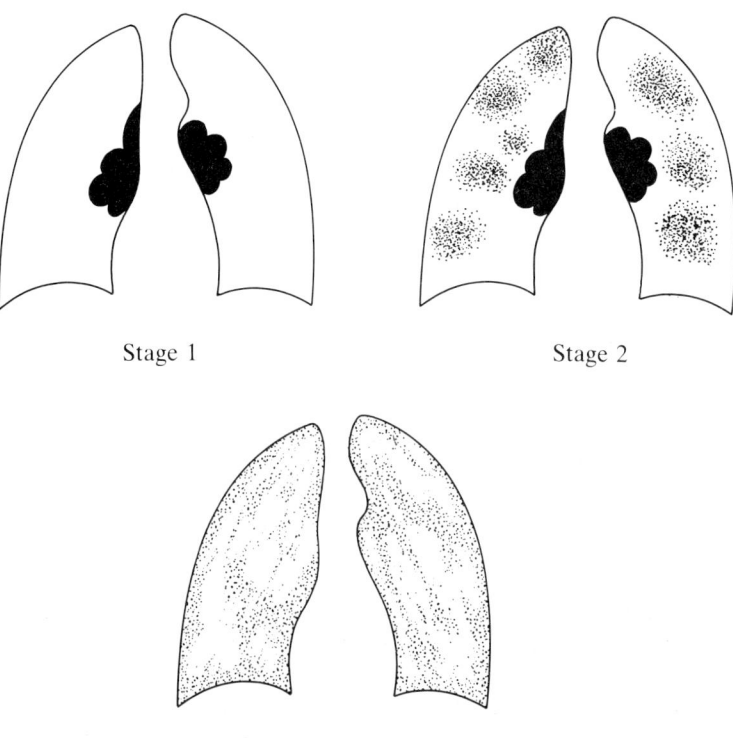

Stage 1   Stage 2

Stage 3

Fig. 17.1 Chest X-ray stages of sarcoidosis. (1) Hilar and mediastinal glandular enlargement, (2) glandular enlargement and pulmonary shadowing, (3) pulmonary shadowing alone (usually widespread).

pulmonary contraction and cystic spaces is sometimes referred to as stage 4.

Hilar glandular disease

Bilateral lymph node enlargement is usually symmetrical and the paratracheal nodes are frequently seen to be involved as well. Very occasionally pulmonary collapse may be caused by compression of bronchi by enlarged glands. The characteristic feature is the symmetrical enlargement of hilar glands which often look like small bunches of grapes (stage 1). Pulmonary shadows may also be present (stage 2).

Pulmonary disease

Pulmonary abnormalities are usually bilateral and widespread. Disseminated miliary or nodular lesions are common, but more confluent shadowing similar to that seen in tuberculosis and pneumonia can also be a manifestation of sarcoidosis (stage 3). Linear shadows extending fan-wise from the hilar regions may be seen and diffuse and patchy areas of abnormality caused by fibrosis are present in chronic cases. Gross pulmonary destruction with cavitation occurs in advanced disease (stage 4).

Investigations

Skin tests. A depressed reaction to antigens with delayed-type hypersensitivity is fairly constantly found in the active phase of sarcoidosis. The simplest and most readily available test is the tuberculin test which is negative in the majority of cases, but a positive tuberculin test does not exclude the diagnosis. The reactions to mumps virus antigen, *Candida albicans* antigen and to trichophytin are also depressed.

Kveim test. The intradermal injection of a particulate saline suspension of sarcoid tissue provokes the slow development of an epithelioid granuloma of sarcoid type. The test should be read at six weeks and histological confirmation of a positive palpable reaction should be obtained by biopsy. This test is positive in the majority of patients with hilar glandular disease, but negative in more than 50% of patients when only the lungs are involved.

Pulmonary function studies. These are normal in hilar glandular disease in the absence of the rare complication of bronchial compression or infiltration. There is poor correlation between the radiological changes and the pulmonary function studies in the early stages of pulmonary sarcoidosis. Frequently no abnormalities can be found in patients with quite extensive pulmonary shadowing. However, fibrosis causes a restrictive defect and impairment of gas transfer. When extensive pulmonary fibrosis has been produced there is gross physiological abnormality including evidence of airways obstruction in some cases.

Differential white cell count. There is often a peripheral blood lymphopenia caused by a reduction in the numbers of T-lymphocytes which produces a relative increase of B-lymphocytes.

Serum globulins may be raised but this is of little diagnostic or prognostic value.

Angiotensin-converting enzyme (ACE) is abnormally high in some patients with sarcoidosis, but serum ACE does not accurately reflect activity of the pulmonary component of the disease as assessed by bronchoalveolar lavage.

Calcium studies. The serum calcium may be elevated in chronic widespread sarcoidosis, but a more common abnormality of calcium metabolism is increased urinary calcium excretion.

Histological confirmation of disease. In patients presenting with pulmonary sarcoidosis the diagnosis often requires to be established histologically, usually by transbronchial biopsy.

Lymph gland biopsy. The glands most often involved are those in the scalene areas which should be biopsied whenever palpable. Mediastinoscopy can be helpful in obtaining biopsies from intrathoracic glands.

Bronchoalveolar lavage (p. 31). Cytological examination of the lavage fluid reveals a high proportion of lymphocytes. There is a close correlation between the intensity of sarcoid alveolitis seen histologically and the proportions of T-lymphocytes in BAL fluid.

Lung biopsy. Transbronchial biopsies obtained via the fibreoptic bronchoscope are often of great value in the investigation of patients with diffuse pulmonary disease. In patients with pulmonary sarcoidosis transbronchial lung biopsy usually confirms the diagnosis, and even when there is only radiographic evidence of hilar and mediastinal glandular involvement a transbronchial lung biopsy often shows typical sarcoid granulomata. Rarely, biopsy at thoracotomy may be necessary.

Biopsy of other tissues. Liver biopsy, skin biopsy and occasionally muscle biopsy may be helpful in some cases.

Sarcoid reaction. The histological demonstration of epithelioid tubercles cannot always be taken as being diagnostic of sarcoidosis. A sarcoid reaction can occur in lymph nodes adjacent to malignant lesions (e.g. lymphomas). Tuberculosis, fungal infections and beryllium disease are also capable of producing non-caseating epithelioid follicles.

Gallium scan (p. 25) can establish the presence of lung inflammation and hence indirectly give information about the activity of pulmonary sarcoidosis, but it is not a specific investigation for sarcoidosis since it is positive in a wide variety of pulmonary disorders.

Differential diagnosis

Although the symmetrical features of glandular sarcoidosis are radiologically characteristic, other causes of mediastinal lymph gland enlargement have to be considered, especially in atypical cases. These include the lymphomas, bronchial carcinoma, primary pulmonary tuberculosis (especially if bilateral) and occasionally pneumonia which can be associated with hilar adenopathy, particularly in Asians.

The differential diagnosis of pulmonary sarcoidosis includes all conditions capable of producing multiple pulmonary shadows, especially tuberculosis, metastatic malignant disease, the pneumoconioses, fibrosing alveolitis, allergic alveolitis and pulmonary eosinophilia.

Treatment

Most patients with glandular sarcoidosis recover spontaneously and therefore require no treatment. Corticosteroid therapy suppresses the formation of sarcoid granulomas and, since it appears likely that granulomatous lesions precede fibrosis, treatment with prednisolone is usually given in an attempt to prevent fibrosis. There is, however, no known cure for this disease and a long-term beneficial effect of corti-costeroid therapy on lung function remains to be proved.

Indications for prednisolone therapy:

1   Pulmonary sarcoidosis associated with a physiological abnormality at the time of diagnosis.
2   Progressive pulmonary sarcoidosis — i.e. deteriorating radiological abnormalities and/or the observed development of functional abnormalities.
3   Persisting or recurring erythema nodosum.
4   Massive glandular sarcoidosis causing bronchial compression.
5   Bronchial sarcoidosis.
6   Extrathoracic sarcoidosis involving vital structures such as the eye, heart and central nervous system.
7   Hypercalcaemia and/or hypercalciuria.

Treatment with prednisolone

Although most cases respond to a relatively small dose of prednisolone (10 mg daily), treatment with an initial daily dose of at least 20 mg should be given for a period of 6–8 weeks to bring the disease under control. Subsequently the dose can be quickly reduced over a period of a few weeks to 10 mg daily. Thereafter the duration of treatment is dependent upon the type of disease being treated. The minimum duration of treatment should be 3–6 months in patients with glandular disease and/or erythema nodosum. In all other cases much more prolonged therapy is necessary. The usual practice is gradually to reduce the dose of prednisolone to below 10 mg daily after a period of about six months. Small reductions in the daily dose of 1 mg every two months can be made with clinical, radiological and physiological checks every 3–4 months. In some cases it is possible to withdraw treatment in this way, but if relapse occurs more prolonged therapy using a dose in excess of that at which relapse occurred should be given. In a few patients life-long therapy has to be given.

The value of serial bronchoalveolar lavage cell counts, gallium scanning and serum angiotensin-converting enzyme estimations is being assessed in respect of the necessity for corticosteroid therapy and also in the monitoring of treatment.

Other drugs such as azathioprine, methotrexate, chlorambucil and chloroquine have been shown to have a suppressive effect on sarcoidosis, but are rarely used because of their potential toxic effects.

Prognosis

Prognosis is usually good since the disease is self-limiting in the majority of cases. Radiographic clearing can be expected within five years in approximately 80% of stage 1 patients and almost 70% of those with stage 2 disease. The prognosis of pulmonary sarcoidosis without hilar glandular enlargement (stage 3) is not as good. Irrespective of treatment, less than half such patients can be expected to have a normal chest X-ray within five years of diagnosis. About 10% of patients initially found to have stage 1 disease will progress to stage 2, and some 15% of stage 2 patients will develop stage 3 radiographs. Progressive pulmonary disease can usually be effectively controlled even though prolonged corticosteroid therapy may be necessary in some cases. Pulmonary fibrosis, however, cannot be reversed with treatment and if this is extensive at the time of diagnosis the prognosis is poor because of the inevitable development of cor pulmonale and respiratory failure.

SUMMARY — SPECIAL POINTS OF EMPHASI

• Erythema nodosum is commonly associated with sarcoidosis.

• The Kveim test is more often positive in patients with hilar glandular enlargement than in other types of sarcoidosis.

• The tuberculin test is often negative.

• Transbronchial lung biopsy is a useful technique in establishing pathological confirmation of the diagnosis of sarcoidosis.

• Bronchoalveolar lavage yields a high proportion of lymphocytes in the lavage fluid in the presence of an active sarcoid alveolitis.

• Gallium scanning and measurement of serum angiotensin-converting enzyme may be useful in the assessment of disease activity.

• Respiratory symptoms are uncommon unless pulmonary involvement has caused extensive fibrosis.

• Abnormal findings on clinical examination usually indicate gross pulmonary fibrosis.

• Sarcoid granulomas in the nasal mucosa frequently are present in patients with intrathoracic sarcoidosis.

• The typical radiological abnormality in glandular sarcoidosis is symmetrical hilar glandular enlargement.

• Hypercalcaemia and hypercalciuria are found only in chronic sarcoidosis.

• Most patients recover spontaneously.

• Corticosteroid therapy readily suppresses the formation of sarcoid granulomas and is indicated in progressive pulmonary disease, especially when there is also evidence of deteriorating pulmonary function, or when other vital organs are affected.

Further reading

Chrétien J., Marsac J. & Laltiel J.C. (Eds.) (1983) *Sarcoidosis and other Granulomatous Disorders.* Oxford: Pergamon Press.

Fanburg B.L. (1983) *Lung Biology in Health and Disease.* Vol. 20, *Sarcoidosis and Other Granulomatous Diseases of the Lung.* New York: Marcel Dekker Inc.

James D.J. & Studdy P.R. (1981) *A Colour Atlas of Respiratory Disease.* London: Wolfe Medical Publications.

Scadding J.G. & Mitchell D.N. (1985) *Sarcoidosis,* 2nd Edition. London: Chapman & Hall.

Simmons D.H. (Ed.) (1981) *Current Pulmonology,* Vol. 3. New York: John Wiley & Sons.

Chapter 18
Adult respiratory distress syndrome

General considerations

Adult respiratory distress syndrome (ARDS) has many causes and may not be a single clinical entity. The common feature is an extensive abnormality in the peripheral, gas-exchanging portions of the lung which causes type I respiratory failure. Injury to the interstitial parts of the lung can result from numerous insults, either via the airways or through the circulation, and hence ARDS can be associated with a wide range of local and systemic disorders (see Table 18.1). There is usually damage to the alveolar epithelium and capillary endothelium which results in the lung tissue becoming flooded with oedema of high protein content. Hypoxaemia may also be caused by alveolar closure secondary to narrowing of the small airways, loss of activity of surfactant and fibrin and platelet microemboli. All non-cardiac causes of pulmonary oedema could be labelled ARDS, and even pulmonary oedema of cardiac origin, especially when associated with hypotension, can lead to ARDS.

There is usually a latent period of 12–48 hours between the initial insult and onset of respiratory symptoms. The cause of death is usually 'multiorgan failure' together with respiratory failure.

It has been suggested that complement-activated polymorphonuclear leucocytes are responsible for the lung lesion in ARDS. An acute fall in white cell count could herald the onset of problems in high-risk patients.

Fundamental points of diagnosis

Respiratory distress is present in all patients. Hyperventilation, hypotension and hypoxaemia is the diagnostic triad, if associated with radiographic pulmonary shadowing. Widespread crepitations, in the absence of evidence of cardiac failure, are audible on auscultation over both lungs. Arterial blood gas analysis in the earlier stages of the syndrome shows type I respiratory failure which becomes severe if the syndrome progresses. Carbon dioxide retention, together with hypoxaemia (type II respiratory failure) occurs as a preterminal event, if mechanical ventilation is not instituted. The chest X-ray shows extensive bilateral pulmonary shadowing caused by interstitial oedema.

Since ARDS has so many causes an attempt must always be made to

Table 18.1 Some causes of adult respiratory distress syndrome.

Pneumonias
Viral
Bacterial
Tuberculosis
Fungal
Pneumocystis carinii
Mycoplasma pneumoniae

Inhaled toxic substances
Corrosive chemicals (ammonia, chlorine, nitrogen dioxide)
High concentrations of oxygen
Smoke

Aspiration of irritant substances
Vomit
Water (fresh and salt water)
Hydrocarbons

Systemic disorders
Shock of any aetiology
Septicaemia
Eclampsia
Uraemia

Blood disorders
Disseminated intravascular coagulation
Thrombotic thrombocytopenic purpura
Massive blood transfusion

Lung emboli
Fat emboli
Air emboli
Amniotic fluid embolism
Lymphangiography

Lung trauma
Lung contusion
Irradiation

Drugs
Diamorphine, methadone, barbiturates, hydrochlorothiazide

Miscellaneous
Post-cardiopulmonary bypass
Increased intracranial pressure
Ascent to high altitudes
Acute pancreatitis

determine the primary condition, since when this is known therapeutic decisions are much easier. It could, however, be argued that the term adult respiratory distress syndrome should be confined to those cases in which a precise pathogenesis is unclear, to avoid an injudicious blanket approach to the diagnosis and management of patients with hypotension, hyperventilation and hypoxaemia associated with a chest X-ray abnormality.

Clinical findings

The clinical presentation of ARDS can be divided into four phases:

1 Breathlessness associated with hypotension, hypoxaemia and respiratory alkalosis. At this time there may be no auscultatory findings, and the chest X-ray may be normal or only show a fine reticular shadowing.

2 Marked respiratory distress because of hyperventilation. Hypotension persists and the hypoxaemia and respiratory alkalosis worsen. Crepitations are audible over both lungs and the X-ray is always abnormal showing bilateral 'soft' shadowing of interstitial pulmonary oedema. These abnormalities are in the absence of any clinical evidence of cardiac failure.

3 Profound respiratory distress and hypoxaemia. The chest X-ray shows extensive bilateral pulmonary shadowing ('bilateral white-out') but the costophrenic angles tend to escape. Numerous crepitations are audible and hypotension is severe. Mechanical ventilation via a cuffed endotracheal tube to allow intermittent positive-pressure ventilation (IPPV) is usually started at this stage. Without artificial ventilation most patients die.

4 Hypoxaemic cardiac arrest, or death from hypoxaemia complicated preterminally by carbon dioxide retention (type II respiratory failure) if not treated by mechanical ventilation. Death from the same causes also occurs in some patients treated by IPPV.

Symptoms and signs

The onset of ARDS should be suspected in all patients with hyperventilation and hypotension (*see* Table 18.1). The patient may be healthy before the onset of symptoms (e.g. prior to inhalation of a toxic substance, aspiration of vomit or embolism of amniotic fluid, etc.) or may be already ill with pneumonia, septicaemia or eclampsia, etc. The prognosis is mainly determined by the cause, but the earlier the diagnosis is made, and appropriate treatment started, the better the prospects of survival. Breathlessness and low blood pressure may be the only clinical abnormalities in the early stages, but widespread crepitations quickly become audible over both lungs. Characteristically these crepitations are present without evidence of cardiac failure. As the syndrome progresses breathlessness becomes more distressing, hypotension persists or gets worse and clinical evidence of hypoxaemia becomes more evident. All patients not severely anaemic become obviously cyanosed. They remain alert and distressed until the terminal stages of carbon dioxide retention and respiratory acidosis.

Radiological examination

In the early stages the X-ray may be only slightly abnormal with a diffuse, but widespread, reticular shadowing, or may simply show the initial pulmonary insult which has led to ARDS, e.g. pneumonia. When the syndrome becomes established, however, chest X-ray shows gross bilateral abnormalities. This extensive pulmonary shadowing is often described as 'soft', 'fluffy' or 'cotton wool'. In advanced cases very little normal lung can be seen and there is almost total 'white-out' of both lung fields, but the costophrenic angles often remain clear.

Investigations

Arterial blood gas analysis which confirms type I respiratory failure is the most important investigation, particularly in assessing response to treatment.

WHITE CELL COUNT

A sudden fall in white cell count may herald the onset of this syndrome. Frequent estimations of WCC in high-risk patients are, therefore, advised.

However, because of the numerous causes of this syndrome (Table 18.1) other investigations (haematological, bacterial, viral, mycological and biochemical) have to be performed, especially when there is doubt why the patient developed ARDS.

Differential diagnosis

The list of differential diagnoses is long, since it includes all causes of type I respiratory failure associated with an abnormal chest X-ray and hypotension. Pulmonary oedema of cardiac origin is high on the list, but all types of pneumonia (not complicated by ARDS), pulmonary thromboembolic disease and most of the other causes of acute type I respiratory failure (p. 78) have to be considered.

Treatment

The treatment priorities of ARDS are:

1 Treatment of the primary disorder.
2 Correction of hypoxaemia.
3 Other measures.

Treatment of the primary disorder

The precipitating condition must, of course, be treated whenever it has been recognized, e.g. pneumonia, septicaemia, etc. However, in most cases the primary disorder is not apparent, and even when it is ARDS can develop in spite of adequate treatment.

Correction of hypoxaemia

Hypoxaemia is a major problem and oxygen in high concentration should be given by face mask. Unfortunately, it is often not possible to maintain an adequate arterial oxygen tension (above 9·0 kPa or 70 mmHg) by this means. In many cases treatment with intermittent positive-pressure ventilation (IPPV) via a cuffed endotracheal tube using a volume-cycled ventilator has to be started at an early stage. Positive end-expiratory pressure (PEEP) is applied to increase the transmural distending pressure across the alveolus in an attempt to reopen alveoli and possibly mechanically decrease pulmonary oedema. Oxygen-enriched air is used to ventilate these patients, the concentration of oxygen being adjusted to maintain a PaO_2 of over 9·0 kPa (70 mmHg) if possible. Prolonged ventilation with very high oxygen concentrations may make the situation worse in that oxygen toxicity can itself cause ARDS. However, in reality as much oxygen as is required to maintain an adequate PaO_2 has to be given and the dangers of oxygen toxicity ignored.

Other measures

TREATMENT OF HYPOTENSION

Patients with ARDS cannot be satisfactorily managed without a central venous pressure line. Hypovolaemia should be promptly corrected but great care must be taken to avoid fluid overload, since this could cause pulmonary oedema and aggravate the pulmonary problems. The question of whether colloid or crystalloid solutions are preferable for volume repletion is still in dispute.

CORTICOSTEROID THERAPY

It is customary to give high-dose corticosteroid therapy, although the value of the treatment is unproven. Intravenous methylprednisolone 1 g daily or 30 mg/kg is often used.

DIURETIC THERAPY

Intravenous frusemide (or equivalent) should be used in all patients with evidence of fluid overload. Experimentally it has been shown that this drug decreases intrapulmonary shunting by a mechanism which is apparently independent of any effect it has on pulmonary arterial wedge pressure. However, overzealous use of diuretics should be avoided because of the risks of creating hypovolaemia.

Prognosis

The prognosis of patients with ARDS of sufficient severity to require mechanical ventilation is poor. At least 50% of patients die in spite of mechanical support. Extracorporeal membrane oxygenation may improve the prognosis in the future. However, many patients may develop less fulminating forms of this syndrome and respond to treatment of the primary condition, without a diagnosis of ARDS being considered. It is, therefore, difficult to estimate the true overall prognosis. The cause of death in ARDS is usually multiorgan failure and not simply respiratory failure.

SUMMARY — SPECIAL POINTS OF EMPHASIS

- ARDS has numerous causes and may not be a single entity.

- High protein-containing fluid in the alveoli and respiratory bronchioles is responsible for type I respiratory failure.

- Multiorgan dysfunction is common in ARDS.

- A fall in peripheral blood white cell count may occur immediately before the onset of ARDS.

- The chest X-ray usually shows extensive bilateral confluent pulmonary shadowing, but in the early stages the costophrenic angles tend to be spared.

- Treatment is of the primary disorder plus correction of hypoxaemia, hypotension and the consequences of multiorgan dysfunction.

- Intermittent positive-pressure ventilation (IPPV) with positive end-expiratory pressure (PEEP) is necessary for the treatment of severely hypoxaemic patients.

- Prognosis is poor if hypoxaemia is severe enough to require artificial ventilation, since less than 50% survive.

Further reading

Boggis C.R.M. & Greene R. (1983) Adult respiratory distress syndrome. *Brit. J. Hosp. Med.* **29**, 167–74.

Cooper T.J. & Tinkler J. (1984) The adult respiratory distress syndrome. *Hospital Update* **10**, 849–59.

Matthay M.A. & Hopewell P.C. (1981) The adult respiratory distress syndrome: pathogenesis and treatment. In *Current Pulmonology, Vol. 3.* (Ed. Simmons D.H.). New York: John Wiley & Sons.

Chapter 19
Miscellaneous conditions

PRIMARY PULMONARY HYPERTENSION

The clinical features of primary pulmonary hypertension are similar to those of thromboembolic pulmonary hypertension but without previous history of thromboembolic phenomena. In Britain pulmonary thrombo-embolism and veno-occlusive disease are the main differential diagnoses, but cardiac causes of secondary pulmonary hypertension have always to be excluded. The chronic bronchopulmonary diseases which cause pulmonary hypertension rarely create diagnostic difficulties, but in tropical countries pulmonary bilharziasis can closely simulate primary pulmonary hypertension. Most patients with this disease are women of child-bearing age, and like thromboembolic pulmonary hypertension it is usually severe by the time symptoms develop.

Chest X-ray often shows a normal-sized heart but with a dilated main pulmonary artery trunk and sometimes increased transradiancy of the lung fields caused by narrowing of peripheral pulmonary vessels.

Electrocardiogram. The ECG usually shows sinus rhythm with right axis deviation and almost invariably T-wave inversion in the right-sided chest leads.

Right heart catheterization reveals a high pulmonary artery pressure, frequently at or about systemic level, when the disease is first recognized.

Pulmonary angiography shows normal anatomy but with dilated proximal branches and attenuation of peripheral small vessels.

Pulmonary veno-occlusive disease

Pulmonary arterial hypertension may develop secondary to thrombotic occlusion of pulmonary veins and venules. This form of secondary pulmonary hypertension occurs at any age, but is more common in childhood and pursues a more rapid course than the primary form. In contrast to primary pulmonary hypertension in which the chest X-ray show hypertranslucent lung fields the chest X-ray in pulmonary veno-occlusive disease shows pulmonary shadowing which may look like pulmonary oedema with septal lines and also pleural effusions. However, there is no evidence of venous distension or inversion of regional flow. There is no known treatment which influences the rapidly fatal course of pulmonary veno-occlusive disease.

The aetiology of primary pulmonary hypertension is unknown, but it is likely that there is more than one cause. There appears, from its sex and age distribution, to be an association with pregnancy or female sex hormones. A familial tendency has been reported, and association with Raynaud's phenomenon, systemic lupus erythematosus, 'mixed connective tissue disease' and hepatic cirrhosis has been described. Pulmonary microembolism, in contrast to the macroembolism seen in thromboembolic pulmonary hypertension, has been postulated as a cause, but this is thought to be unlikely.

Drugs and pulmonary hypertension

An 'epidemic' of pulmonary hypertension in Switzerland, a few years ago, was attributed to the use of the slimming drug aminorex fumarate, and recently the chemically related drug fenfluramine has also been incriminated. Other drugs which may cause pulmonary hypertension are listed in Table 19.1.

Table 19.1 Some causes of pulmonary hypertension.

Primary pulmonary hypertension
Thromboembolic pulmonary hypertension
Pulmonary veno-occlusive disease
Pulmonary bilharziasis

Cardiac disorders. Left ventricular failure, mitral valve disease, left atrial tumour, congenital anomalies of pulmonary veins, congenital septal defects, etc.

Chronic bronchopulmonary diseases. Chronic bronchitis, bronchiectasis, tuberculosis, sarcoidosis, fibrosing alveolitis, etc.

Connective tissue diseases. Systemic lupus erythematosus, 'mixed connective tissue disease', scleroderma, Raynaud's phenomenon, etc.

Drugs. Aminorex fumarate, fenfluramine, chlorphentermine, phenformin, oral contraceptives.

Others. High altitude (Monge's disease), hepatic cirrhosis, lung irradiation in infancy.

Treatment

Treatment of pulmonary hypertension is generally unsatisfactory. Drugs should, of course, be withdrawn, since drug-induced pulmonary hypertension is often reversible. Treatment with diazoxide, hydrallazine or nifedipine should be tried, since occasionally there is dramatic response or even remission. Spontaneous improvement also sometimes occurs, but usually the clinical course from the onset of symptoms is relentless progression to death within 2–10 years.

DRUG-INDUCED RESPIRATORY DISORDERS

Drugs can affect the respiratory system in many different ways:

1 By their specific pharmacological actions.
2 By inducing allergic reactions in the bronchi and/or lungs.
3 By producing diffuse pulmonary disease affecting alveoli and aveolar walls which usually results in pulmonary fibrosis.
4 By inducing a systemic lupus erythematosus-like syndrome with pulmonary and pleural changes.
5 By exposing patients to opportunistic pulmonary infection as a consequence of therapeutic immunosuppression.
6 By disturbing the normal mechanisms of coagulation and causing either thromboembolic disease or bronchopulmonary haemorrhage.
7 By producing localized or diffuse bronchopulmonary lesions when inhaled accidentally or as a diagnostic or therapeutic measure.

1 Specific pharmacological effects

Bronchoconstriction can be induced in asthmatic patients by beta-adrenoreceptor blocking drugs, and even the 'cardioselective' drugs should be avoided, or used with extreme caution, in patients with asthma or chronic obstructive bronchitis.

Cholinergic drugs (e.g. methacholine, carbachol, etc.) cause broncho-constriction by parasympathetic stimulation. Methacholine inhalation is used deliberately to induce bronchoconstriction under laboratory conditions in order to assess bronchial reactivity (bronchial challenge test).

Central respiratory depression produced by opiates and all sedative drugs can lead to type II respiratory failure, particularly in patients with severe chronic bronchitis.

2 Allergic reactions

Bronchoconstriction and pulmonary eosinophilia can be manifestations of drug allergy. Bronchospasm is also a feature of more generalized anaphylactic reactions. Protein-containing preparations such as antisera and vaccines are particularly prone to cause allergic reactions (usually bronchoconstriction). It has been well known for many years that aspirin can provoke asthma, but since this is likely to be due to its pharmacological effect upon prostaglandin synthesis, it cannot be regarded as a true allergic response. Other non-steroidal anti-inflammatory drugs (NSAIDs) also precipitate attacks in asthmatics. It is by no means clear why some drugs cause asthmatic reactions and others pulmonary eosinophilia.

Some preparations known to cause asthma are:
Penicillin and other antibiotics
Aspirin and other NSAIDs
Monoamine oxidase inhibitors
Antisera and some vaccines
Allergen extracts used for hyposensitization
Blood and blood products
i.v. contrast media used in X-ray diagnosis.

Some of the drugs known to cause pulmonary eosinophilia are:
Nitrofurantoin
Para-aminosalicylic acid
Sulphonamides
Imipramine
Chlorpropamide
Phenylbutazone
Aspirin
Penicillin and other antibiotics
Methotrexate.

3 Diffuse pulmonary disease

This is a heterogenous group of reactions which range from florid alveolitis histologically mimicking adenocarcinoma to pulmonary reactions resembling ARDS (p. 271). Cytotoxic drugs such as bleomycin and busulphan are more likely to give problems in patients who have received therapeutic pulmonary irradiation.

Some of the drugs known to cause diffuse pulmonary reaction without eosinophilia are:

Bleomycin
Busulphan
Melphalan
Cyclophosphamide
Methotrexate
Mitomycin C
Gold
Pindolol
Amiodarone
Antazoline.

4 Systemic lupus erythematosus-like syndrome

A syndrome closely resembling systemic lupus erythematosus is known to be produced by drugs such as hydrallazine, procainamide, isoniazid and phenytoin. Recovery is usual after stopping the offending drug, but permanent pleural thickening and pulmonary fibrosis can occur, particularly if there is delay in drug withdrawal.

5 Opportunistic pulmonary infection

Pulmonary infection in the immunocompromised patient is a serious and increasing problem (see p. 106).

6 Coagulation disorders

Oestrogen-containing oral contraceptives predispose to pulmonary thromboembolism. Bronchopulmonary bleeding can result from cytotoxic chemotherapy-induced thrombocytopenia and, of course, from poorly controlled anticoagulant therapy.

7 Focal and diffuse pulmonary lesions caused by inhalation

Lipoid pneumonia can result from inhalation of liquid paraffin, particularly in patients with oesophageal abnormalities causing hold-up (e.g. achalasia). Iodine-containing opaque media suspended in arachis oil used for bronchography may produce lipoid granuloma and more florid pulmonary reactions requiring corticosteroid treatment.

OTHER IATROGENIC PULMONARY PROBLEMS

Pulmonary oedema may be induced by i.v. fluid overload, narcotic drug overdosage, cardiopulmonary angiographic procedures and by drugs.

Pleural fibrosis occurs occasionally in patients being treated for migraine with methysergide, and this complication was the reason why oral practolol was withdrawn. Acebutolol has recently been incriminated as a cause of recurrent pleurisy, together with pulmonary granulomatous disease.

Oxygen in high concentration can cause pulmonary damage which can progress to ARDS (p. 271). Oxygen can, of course, cause central depression of respiratory drive in patients with type II respiratory failure.

Aminoglycoside antibiotics may potentiate the action of muscle relaxant drugs and occasionally themselves cause neuromuscular weakness in uraemic patients.

Iatrogenic bronchopulmonary disease is common and often overlooked. In all patients with respiratory problems detailed information about current and recent drug treatment should be listed and the possibility of a drug-induced disorder should be constantly kept in mind. Pulmonary hypertension may be drug-induced (p. 279).

PULMONARY EOSINOPHILIA

Definition: a group of diseases differing in aetiology but having two common features:

(a)   Transient pulmonary opacities on chest X-ray.
(b)   An increased peripheral blood eosinophil count.

There is no satisfactory classification of these disorders, but it is useful to divide them into two main groups:

1   Pulmonary eosinophilia with asthma.
2   Pulmonary eosinophilia without asthma.

1   Pulmonary eosinophilia with asthma (p. 119)

In approximately 60% of these patients with asthma the pulmonary disorder is due to hypersensitivity to *Aspergillus fumigatus,* probably involving a combination of type I and type III hypersensitivity reactions. In the remaining patients the cause is unknown.

2   Pulmonary eosinophilia without asthma

CAUSES KNOWN

1   Helminths, e.g. ascaris, toxocara, filaria.
2   Drugs, e.g. nitrofurantoin, PAS, antibiotics (*see* p. 281).
3   Fungi, especially *A. fumigatus.*
4   Polyarteritis nodosa (rare).

CAUSE UNKNOWN

Eosinophilic pneumonia (cryptogenic pulmonary eosinophilia)

This may be a benign form of polyarteritis nodosa. It is characterized by an acute febrile illness associated with gross elevation of the ESR, a very high blood eosinophil count and pulmonary radiographic shadowing. The X-ray abnormalities which may be extensive and confluent are most often peripherally situated in the upper lobes and frequently look like tuberculosis. This type of pulmonary eosinophilia does not give rise to bronchiectasis.

Treatment.   There is usually dramatic response to prednisolone, X-ray clearing occurring within a few days of treatment with 20 mg daily. In some patients a gradual withdrawal of therapy is possible without recurrence but a small maintenance dose of 5 mg daily or even less may be necessary to suppress the disease.

RESPIRATORY MANIFESTATIONS OF CONNECTIVE TISSUE DISEASES

Systemic lupus erythematosus

Pleural effusion, which is often bilateral and accompanied by pericardial effusion, is a relatively common manifestation of systemic lupus erythematosus. Rapidly progressing fibrosing alveolitis which, however, usually responds well to corticosteroid therapy is also a manifestation of this disease. Patchy areas of 'lupus pneumonitis' may also be seen on X-ray, and are probably caused by arteritis and superimposed bacterial infection.

Polyarteritis nodosa

This is said to be one of the causes of pulmonary eosinophilia without asthma (*see above*). Pulmonary hypertension may result from intimal fibrosis of arteries and arterioles. Wegener's granulomatosis, which is probably a variant of polyarteritis nodosa, causes granulomatous lesions in the lungs, resulting in multiple X-ray shadows.

Systemic sclerosis

Fibrosing alveolitis which does not respond well to corticosteroid therapy is the most common respiratory manifestation of systemic sclerosis. Pulmonary hypertension may result from intimal fibrosis of arteries and arterioles.

Dermatomyositis

Fibrosing alveolitis may be associated with dermatomyositis. Weakness of intercostal muscles and the diaphragm sometimes leads to respiratory failure and aspiration pneumonia. Laryngeal muscle weakness, causing hoarseness, can also predispose to aspiration pneumonia. In a proportion of patients with dermatomyositis there is an associated malignant disease which is often bronchial carcinoma.

Rheumatoid disease

There are many respiratory manifestations of rheumatoid disease, which include:

Pleural effusion, which is more common in males and usually chronic, and may, therefore, contain cholesterol crystals (p. 169). Pleural friction and pleural thickening may occur without effusion.

Fibrosing alveolitis (rheumatoid lung) (p. 212). The rate of progression is variable. Response to treatment with corticosteroids is usually poor.

Pulmonary rheumatoid nodules. These may be single or multiple and vary greatly in size. Usually nodules are subpleural and if cavitation occurs may cause pneumothorax. In patients with pneumoconiosis (e.g. coalworker's pneumoconiosis or asbestosis) the development of pulmonary rheumatoid nodules is often referred to as Caplan's syndrome. Pulmonary nodules usually develop in patients with sub-cutaneous rheumatoid nodules.

Pulmonary vascular changes are uncommon but pulmonary hyper-tension and obliterative arteritis occasionally occur.

Cricoaretenoid arthritis may cause weakness of the voice and reduce movement of the vocal cords, leading to laryngeal obstruction in some cases.

Pulmonary fibrosis. Upper lobe fibrosis similar to that found in ankylosing spondylitis (p. 293) may also occur in rheumatoid disease.

Bronchopulmonary bacterial infection occurs more frequently in patients with rheumatoid disease than normal individuals.

Airways obstruction. About one-third of patients with rheumatoid disease can be shown to have evidence of air flow obstruction.

Obliterative bronchiolitis is a rare but distressing complication of rheumatoid disease. Progressive breathlessness is the presenting symptom and end-inspiratory 'squeaks' are easily audible on auscultation. The chest X-ray is often normal.

Tuberculosis. Corticosteroid therapy used to control joint symptoms can predispose to the development of pulmonary tuberculosis. The diagnosis may be overlooked at an early stage because of the assumption that the X-ray changes are caused by one of the specific respiratory manifestations of rheumatoid disease.

Rheumatic fever

A slowly resolving fibrinoid pneumonia may develop in patients with rheumatic fever.

Diagnosis

Diagnosis of the connective tissue disorder is usually made from the non-respiratory manifestations of the disease, supported by elevation of the ESR, and serological tests (antinuclear factor, LE cells, rheumatoid factor).

Treatment

The treatment of respiratory manifestations of connective tissue diseases is generally unsatisfactory, but corticosteroid therapy should be tried in progressive lesions such as fibrosing alveolitis. Usually, response is poor except in patients with systemic lupus erythematosus. Azathioprine combined with prednisolone may be effective in some cases and should be tried in patients with polyarteritis nodosa. Cyclophosphamide and prednisolone is the treatment of choice for Wegener's granulomatosis. Occasionally it may be wise to give antituberculosis therapy in conjunction with corticosteroids if there is significant diagnostic doubt.

IDIOPATHIC PULMONARY HAEMOSIDEROSIS

General considerations

This is a rare disease of children and young adults characterized by recurrent intrapulmonary haemorrhage, the deposition of haemosiderin in the lungs, and the development of interstitial pulmonary fibrosis.

Fundamental points of diagnosis

Recurrent episodes of haemoptysis associated with pulmonary X-ray shadowing and anaemia.

Complications

Death may occur from massive intrapulmonary haemorrhage. Pulmonary fibrosis often leads to death from cor pulmonale and respiratory failure.

Clinical findings

Symptoms and signs

Recurrent episodes of haemoptysis associated with breathlessness and pallor are the classical symptoms. Progressive breathlessness occurs with the development of widespread pulmonary fibrosis. There are often no abnormal clinical signs on examination except for clinical evidence of anaemia. Crepitations may be audible over areas of pulmonary haemorrhage. Finger clubbing occurs in about 25% of patients.

Radiological examination

During episodes of intrapulmonary haemorrhage the X-ray may show blotchy pulmonary shadows or areas of confluent shadowing. When pulmonary fibrosis has developed diffuse pulmonary stippling can be seen, especially in the mid and lower zones. Enlargement of mediastinal lymph nodes is not uncommon.

Investigations

Sputum. Haemosiderin-containing macrophages are usually abundant in sputum or gastric washings.

Blood. Iron deficiency anaemia is present except during prolonged remissions.

Lung biopsy may have to be performed in some cases. This shows intra-alveolar haemorrhage with haemosiderin-containing macrophages in alveolar spaces and alveolar walls, with varying degrees of alveolar septal fibrosis. Haemosiderin-containing macrophages are seen in bronchoalveolar lavage specimens.

Differential diagnosis

This disease has to be differentiated from Goodpasture's disease. In adults the disease is often initially thought to be pulmonary infarction.

Treatment

Many treatments including corticosteroids and azathioprine have been tried but it has not yet been established whether any treatment is of benefit. Blood transfusion may be necessary during severe episodes.

Prognosis

The prognosis is extremely variable. The disease is usually fatal but some patients have long periods of remission.

GOODPASTURE'S DISEASE

Intrapulmonary haemorrhage giving rise to clinical features similar to those of idiopathic pulmonary haemosiderosis can affect young adults, especially males, and occur in association with glomerulonephritis. In some patients the haemoptysis will predate renal symptoms by months or even years; others will present with a nephrotic syndrome, haematuria, or even oliguric renal failure. In all the urine will contain protein, red cells and red cell casts. The condition is associated with the production of anti-glomerular basement membrane antibody and occurs most frequently in subjects who are HLA DR2. A history of preceding upper respiratory tract infection is quite common. This disease is usually fatal but encouraging results have been achieved with plasmaphaeresis.

A similar syndrome (Goodpasture's syndrome) may be produced by reactions to drugs such as penicillamine.

CYSTIC FIBROSIS

General considerations

Cystic fibrosis is a hereditary disorder (autosomal recessive gene) characterized by pancreatic insufficiency, chronic bronchopulmonary infection and high sweat electrolyte concentrations. Most of the pathological changes in this disease are due to mucus obstruction of mucus-secreting glands. It is relatively common in Caucasian children, occurring in approximately 1:2000 live births, but rare in Negroes and Orientals. Respiratory symptoms develop in most cases in early infancy but the diagnosis may be first made in adolescence or early adult life.

Fundamental points of diagnosis

The disease should be suspected in children and young adults who have recurrent or chronic bronchopulmonary infection, especially if there is also evidence of pancreatic insufficiency. The only reliable diagnostic test is the quantitative sweat test.

Complications

Chronic or recurrent bronchopulmonary infection gives rise to bronchiectasis, pulmonary fibrosis and death at an early age from ventilatory failure and cor pulmonale.

Clinical findings

Symptoms and signs

In the early stages there may be recurrent episodes of cough, purulent sputum and wheeze, but cough quickly becomes chronic and wheeze and breathlessness progressive. Sputum is frequently purulent and may be copious.

There may be few abnormal signs in the early stages, but progressive pulmonary destruction results in the signs of bronchiectasis and chronic airways obstruction. Hepatosplenomegaly may be present. The general nutrition of the patient may be poor and growth retarded. Finger clubbing is common when chronic bronchial infection has become established. In the terminal stages there may be cyanosis and evidence of cor pulmonale.

Radiological examination

The chest X-ray may be normal initially or simply show evidence of acute pulmonary infection. As the disease progresses destruction of bronchopulmonary architecture occurs, especially in the upper lobes. Hyperinflation of the lungs is a common finding.

Investigations

Sweat test. The pilocarpine iontophoresis method of collecting sweat is the easiest and most reliable test. At least 50 mg of sweat is necessary for accurate analysis. The finding of a sweat sodium level of above 70 mmol/l in children strongly supports a diagnosis of cystic fibrosis. However, this test is unreliable in adults.

Pancreatic function studies may have to be performed in some patients.

Sputum. Frequent bacteriological examination of sputum is important. *Staphylococcus pyogenes* and *Pseudomonas aeruginosa* are frequent pathogens. Bronchial colonization with *A. fumigatus* occurs in a high proportion of patients surviving into adult life.

Differential diagnosis

The differential diagnosis includes all causes of repeated or chronic bronchopulmonary infections in young patients such as bronchiectasis and the rare condition of primary hypogammaglobulinaemia. Sometimes cystic fibrosis has to be excluded in children who have repeated bronchial infections associated with asthma.

Treatment

There is no specific therapy. Treatment is aimed at the prevention and control of pulmonary infection.

Physiotherapy. In acute infections postural drainage and chest wall percussion is of value. When bronchiectasis has developed regular postural drainage should be performed (p. 52).

Antibiotic therapy. Antibiotic therapy is essential in the treatment of acute infective exacerbations. Sputum should always be examined bacteriologically and appropriate changes of antibiotic therapy made according to the results of culture and antibiotic sensitivity tests. *Staph. aureus* is a common pathogen and when present potent antistaphylococcal agents should be used (*see* p. 103).

Long-term antibiotic treatment is avoided by some physicians because of the risks of creating antibiotic-resistant organisms or encouraging bronchial colonization with Gram-negative bacteria. It is, however, probably advisable to continue treatment of acute exacerbations for 6–8 weeks in an attempt to eradicate bacterial infections completely and avoid rapid recurrence of infection.

Pseudomonas aeruginosa is frequently cultured from sputum of patients with gross pulmonary destruction. When the patient is acutely ill treatment with a drug such as gentamicin (5–6 mg/kg body weight daily, i.v. or i.m.), tobramycin (3–5 mg/kg body weight daily, i.v. or i.m.) and/or azlocillin (2–5 g i.v. eight-hourly) should be considered. Ceftazidime (1–6 g i.v. daily) appears to offer considerable promise in the treatment of troublesome pseudomonas infection. When chronic bronchial infection is not associated with systemic upset antibiotic therapy is probably best avoided.

Aerosol therapy. Antibiotics and mucolytic drugs are often administered by aerosol using a Wright nebulizer and compressor unit or oxygen supply. The benefits of these treatments are questionable. Bronchodilators and/or saline given by aerosol before physiotherapy may be of help in clearing bronchial secretions.

Domiciliary self- or relative-administered intravenous antibiotic therapy has recently tried with some success. The difficulties of i.v. injections can usually be overcome by appropriate instruction.

Nutrition. It is important to ensure, as far as is possible, good nutrition by dietary management and pancreatic enzyme replacement therapy.

Prognosis

Although the prognosis of cystic fibrosis has improved in recent years, only 25% of patients can be expected to survive to the age 20. Survival does not appear to be related to the age of onset of symptoms. Prolonged survival is rare.

Further reading

Goodchild M.T. & Dodge J.A. (1985) *Cystic Fibrosis: Manual of Diagnosis and Management*, 2nd Edition. Philadelphia: Baillière Tindall.

Grant I.W.B. (1982) Bronchopulmonary eosinophilia. *Hospital Update* **8**, 491–501.

Hodson M.E., Norman A.P. & Batten J.C. (Eds.) (1983) *Cystic Fibrosis* London: Baillière Tindall.

Liebow A.A. & Carrington C.B. (1968) The eosinophilic pneumonias. *Medicine (Baltimore)* **48**, 251–85.

Petrie J.C. (1980) *Clinically Important Adverse Drug Interactions. 1. Cardiovascular and Respiratory Disease Therapy.* Amsterdam: Elsevier/North Holland:

Chapter 20
Abnormalities of the chest wall and diaphragm

ABNORMALITIES OF CHEST WALL SHAPE

Barrel chest (p. 44), *pigeon chest* (p. 13), and *Harrison's sulci* (p. 13) can be the result of long-standing obstructive airways disease.

Pectus excavatum (funnel chest) (p.13) is a developmental abnormality which produces little or no functional abnormality unless depression of the sternum is very marked. This deformity is often cosmetically unacceptable to patients, but surgical treatment is rarely necessary. The PA chest X-ray often shows cardiac displacement to the left.

Kyphosis and kyphoscoliosis

Abnormalities of alignment of the dorsal spine and its consequent effects on thoracic shape may be caused by:

1 Congenital abnormality.
2 Vertebral disease such as tuberculosis, osteoporosis and ankylosing spondylitis.
3 Trauma.
4 Neuromuscular disease such as poliomyelitis.

Kyphosis causes less pulmonary embarrassment than scoliosis. Severe kyphoscoliosis often causes rapidly fatal ventilatory failure at an early age.

Ankylosing spondylitis

Ankylosis of the costovertebral joints causes immobilization of the ribs and loss of chest expansion. Ventilation is then solely dependent upon diaphragm movement. In some cases there is associated kyphosis involving the upper dorsal and cervical vertebrae. Patients with ankylosing spondylitis have a poor prognosis when there is associated chronic obstructive airways disease because of early development of respiratory failure.

Patients with ankylosing spondylitis may develop pulmonary fibrosis, usually in the upper lobes, which may cavitate and become colonized with *Aspergillus fumigatus*. This complication increases breathlessness already present because of rib fixation and is usually slowly progressive. It cannot be distinguished radiologically from tuberculosis, which also may be more common in patients with ankylosing spondylitis than in the normal population.

There is no specific treatment for the respiratory complications of ankylosing spondylitis but all patients should be advised not to smoke because of the poor prognosis produced by the combination of chronic obstructive bronchitis and loss of rib movement.

RIBS

Congenital abnormalities of the ribs are common but of no clinical significance, except in the case of cervical ribs which may produce symptoms of thoracic outlet compression. Abnormalities include bifid ribs, fusion of ribs, extra ribs and absence of ribs. These are usually detected as chance radiological findings.

Fractured ribs may be the result of local trauma, coughing (cough fracture) or malignant lesions, usually metastatic (pathological fracture). The symptoms produced by fractured ribs may be mistaken for pleuritic pain, but acute local tenderness or pain at the fracture site induced by gentle pressure on the sternum (springing of the chest) usually indicates the diagnosis.

Rib fractures may be difficult to detect on the chest X-ray even when special views of the ribs concerned are taken.

TREATMENT OF FRACTURED RIBS

Rib fractures in patients with healthy lungs do not require specific treatment unless there are multiple fractures. If sufficient ribs are fractured to produce a *'flail chest'*, paradoxical chest wall movement will occur with respiration. High concentrations of oxygen should be given and in the most severely injured immediate endotracheal intubation and positive-pressure ventilation will be required. Adhesive strapping to the affected site should be avoided, especially in patients with underlying respiratory disease. Potent analgesic drugs may precipitate respiratory failure in patients with underlying bronchopulmonary disease, and in these patients relief of pain can be achieved by local anaesthesia. Intercostal nerve block or infiltration of the fracture site can effectively relieve pain temporarily, but there is a risk of pneumothorax with these procedures. Epidural analgesia can be used in some patients with severe chronic bronchitis who cannot cough because of pain. There is no curative treatment for pathological fractures due to metastatic disease, but in addition to local anaesthesia palliative radiotherapy can produce pain relief in some patients. Most patients with rib fractures will sleep much more comfortably sitting in a chair than lying down.

Primary tumours and infections of the ribs are rare.

DIAPHRAGM

Diaphragmatic paralysis

Phrenic nerve damage leading to paralysis of the hemidiaphragm is most often produced by bronchial carcinoma (p. 132) but can also be the result of a number of neurological disorders, injury or disease of cervical vertebrae and tumours of the spinal cord. Trauma to the neck, including birth injuries, and stretching of the phrenic nerve by mediastinal masses and aortic aneurysms may also lead to diaphragmatic paralysis. Formerly, deliberate trauma (phrenic crush) was used as a treatment of tuberculosis. Occasionally and inexplicably, phrenic nerve palsy follows pulmonary infarction and very rarely pneumonia. Sometimes no cause is detected.

Paralysis of one hemidiaphragm results in loss of approximately 20% of ventilatory capacity, but this is usually not noticed by patients.

Diagnosis is suggested by elevation of the hemidiaphragm on the PA radiograph and confirmed by screening (p. 145).

Eventration of the diaphragm

This is usually a congenital disorder caused by absence of muscular fibres in the diaphragm. It is more common in males and affects the left hemidiaphragm much more commonly than the right. The hemidiaphragm is elevated on X-ray and may appear thin if outlined by a gas-filled viscus beneath it. Eventrations of the diaphragm move paradoxically on screening (p. 145).

Causes of elevation of a hemidiaphragm

1   Phrenic nerve paralysis.
2   Eventration of the diaphragm.
3   Decrease in volume of the lung, e.g. by lobectomy, unilateral pulmonary fibrosis.

4   Severe pleuritic pain from any cause.
5   Pulmonary   infarction — screening   may   show   paradoxical
movement.
6   Subphrenic abscess.
7   Large volumes of gas in the stomach or colon.
8   Large tumours or cysts of the liver.

Apparent elevation of a hemidiaphragm may be simulated by:

(i)   Subpulmonary collection of fluid.
(ii)   A large mass in the lower lobe.
(iii) Collapse of the right middle and lower lobes (which also causes
hemidiaphragm elevation).

Further reading

James   J.I.P.   (1976)   *Scoliosis*,   2nd   Edition.   Edinburgh: Churchill
    Livingstone.

Chapter 21
Diseases of the mediastinum

ACUTE MEDIASTINITIS

The most common cause of this usually devastating disease which is often accompanied by mediastinal emphysema is rupture of the oesophagus (p. 187).

MEDIASTINAL FIBROSIS

Progressive fibrosis within the mediastinum may be idiopathic or induced by drugs such as practolol and possibly methysergide. The clinical presentation is usually that of superior vena caval obstruction or occlusion of one of its tributaries. Stricture of the trachea or main bronchi, the pulmonary veins and the oesophagus may occur. The chest X-ray may show upper mediastinal widening and there may also be evidence of pleural fibrosis.

MEDIASTINAL MASSES

Mediastinal masses are frequently asymptomatic and detected on routine X-ray. Occasionally the nature of mediastinal lesions may be suggested by associated clinical abnormalities such as myasthenia gravis (thymic tumours), generalized lymphadenopathy (lymphomas) or cardiovascular abnormalities (aortic aneurysm). Increase in size of benign mediastinal lesions may cause symptoms due to mechanical compression of mediastinal structures. Malignant lesions may produce problems because of compression or invasion of structures. Compression of the trachea and main bronchi can produce cough, breathlessness and stridor. Oesophageal compression usually presents with dysphagia. Superior vena caval obstruction is more common with malignant lesions than benign tumours. Laryngeal nerve involvement produces hoarseness and bovine cough. Phrenic nerve damage causes diaphragmatic paralysis. Pain of intercostal nerve distribution may be produced by neurogenic tumours which also can occasionally result in cord compression.

The mediastinum can be divided into four major compartments with reference to the lateral chest X-ray (Fig. 21.1):

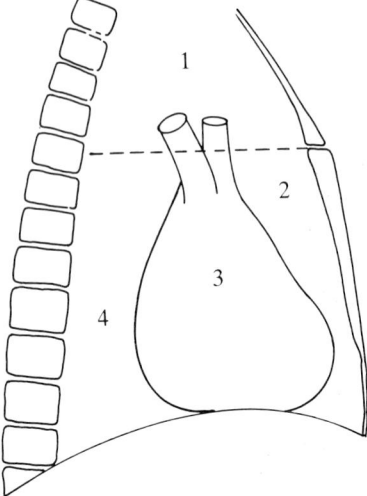

Fig. 21.1   Compartments of the mediastinum.

Superior mediastinum — above a line drawn between the 5th dorsal vertebral body and the upper end of the body of the sternum.

Anterior mediastinum — in front of the heart.

Posterior mediastinum — behind the heart.

Middle mediastinum — between the anterior and posterior compartments.

The most commonly encountered masses in the four compartments are:

Superior mediastinum

1   Retrosternal goitre.
2   Vascular lesions:
      persistent left superior vena cava
      prominent left subclavian artery.
3   Thymic tumours.
4   Dermoid cysts.
5   Lymphomas.
6   Aortic aneurysm.

Anterior mediastinum

1 Retrosternal goitre.
2 Dermoid cysts.
3 Thymic tumours.
4 Lymphomas.
5 Aortic aneurysm.
6 Pericardial cysts.
7 Hernias through the diaphragmatic foramen of Morgagni.

Posterior mediastinum

1 Neurogenic tumours.
2 Paravertebral abscesses.
3 Oesophageal lesions.
4 Aortic aneurysm.
5 Foregut duplications.

Middle mediastinum

1 Bronchial carcinoma.
2 Lymphomas.
3 Sarcoidosis.
4 Bronchogenic cysts.

Investigations

Conventional tomography can be of value in defining the exact site of a mass and also in the detection of calcification within the lesion. Calcification occurs in dermoid cysts, thyroid lesions and less commonly in thymomas.

Computerized axial tomography (CT). Probably the most fruitful use of CT in the investigation of thoracic diseases is in the definition of abnormal mediastinal masses.

Screening may be helpful in the investigation of phrenic nerve involvement and vascular lesions. Pulsation of vascular lesions will be seen but transmitted pulsation from the aorta and main pulmonary arteries is common with solid tumours adjacent to these vessels.

Barium swallow may show narrowing or displacement of the barium outlined oesophageal lumen.

Angiography may be necessary to define accurately aneurysms of the great vessels.

Mediastinoscopy can be of great value in the investigation of many mediastinal masses.

Bronchoscopy is indicated when there is evidence of compression of trachea and/or main bronchi.

Treatment

Single mediastinal masses are often best dealt with by surgical removal because it may not be possible to establish a definite diagnosis before surgical exploration. Radiotherapy is of value in some malignant disorders after the diagnosis has been made by thoracotomy or mediastinoscopy.

Further reading

Davidson K.G., Walbaum P.R. & McCormack R.J.M. (1978) Intrathoracic neural tumours. *Thorax* **33**, 359.

Golding S. (1984) Indications for computed tomography of the chest. *Hospital Update* **10**, 237–51.

Marchevsky A.M. & Kaneko M. (1984) *Surgical Pathology of the Mediastinum*. New York: Raven Press.

Morrison I.M. (1958) Tumours and cysts of the mediastinum. *Thorax* **13**, 294.

Further reading

Clark T.J.H. (Ed.) (1981) *Clinical Investigation of Respiratory Disease.* London: Chapman & Hall.

Cole R.B. (1981) *Drug Treatment of Respiratory Disease.* Edinburgh: Churchill Livingstone.

Cotes J.E. (1979) *Lung Function*, 4th edition. Oxford. Blackwell Scientific Publications.

Crofton J. & Douglas A. (1981) *Respiratory Diseases*, 3rd Edition. Oxford: Blackwell Scientific Publications.

Crompton G.K. (1982) Steroids in respiratory disease. *Brit. J. Hosp. Med.* **28**, 340–8.

Cumming G. & Semple S.J. (1980) *Disorders of the Respiratory System*, 2nd Edition. Oxford: Blackwell Scientific Publications.

Emerson P. (Ed.) (1981) *Thoracic Medicine.* London: Butterworth. Scientific Ltd

Gibson G.J. (1984) *Clinical Tests of Respiratory Function.* New York: Raven Press.

James D.J. & Studdy P.R. (1981) *A Colour Atlas of Respiratory Diseases.* London: Wolfe Medical Publications Ltd.

Macleod J. (Ed.) (1986) *Clinical Examination*, 7th Edition. Edinburgh: Churchill Livingstone.

Morgenroth K., Newhouse M.T. & Nolte D. (1982) *Atlas of Pulmonary Pathology.* London: Butterworth Scientific Ltd.

Simon G. (1978) *Chest X-ray Diagnosis*, 4th Edition. London: Butterworth Scientific Ltd.

Simmons D.H. (Ed.) (1981) *Current Pulmonology.* Vol 3. New York: John Wiley & Sons.

Sterling G.M. (1983) *Integrated Clinical Science Respiratory Disease.* London: Heinemann.

Index